PROZAC
AND OTHER
PSYCHIATRIC
DRUGS

PROZAC
AND OTHER
PSYCHIATRIC
DRUGS

LEWIS A. OPLER, M.D., PH.D.
and CAROL BIALKOWSKI

POCKET BOOKS
New York   London   Toronto   Sydney   Tokyo   Singapore

*Dr. Lewis A. Opler dedicates this book
to his patients, who have taught him much
of what he knows.*

*Carol Bialkowski dedicates this book to her father,
Joseph Bialkowski.*

An *Original* Publication of POCKET BOOKS

POCKET BOOKS, a division of Simon & Schuster Inc.
1230 Avenue of the Americas, New York, NY 10020

Copyright © 1996 by Lynn Sonberg Book Associates

Published by arrangement with:

Lynn Sonberg Book Associates
10 West 86th Street
New York, NY 10024

ISBN: 0-671-51070-3

First Pocket Books printing July 1996

10 9 8 7 6 5 4 3 2 1

POCKET and colophon are registered trademarks of Simon & Schuster Inc.

Cover photo by Jonathan Novrok/Tony Stone Images

Printed in the U.S.A.

Important Note

This book was written to provide selected information to the public concerning frequently prescribed psychiatric medications. Research about prescription drugs is an ongoing process; side effects and adverse reactions to particular drugs sometimes continue to be reported to the FDA after a drug has been approved for use in the general market. While efforts have been made to include up-to-date information in this book, there can be no guarantee that what we know about psychiatric drugs won't change with time and further research. Readers should bear in mind that this book is not intended to be used for self-diagnosis or self-treatment; they should consult appropriate health professionals regarding all psychiatric or medical problems. Readers should never stop taking a prescription drug or alter the dosage or dosing schedule without first consulting their physicians. Neither the publisher, the producer, nor the authors take any responsibility for any possible consequences from any treatment, action, or application of medicine or preparation by any person reading or following the information in this book.

Please note that the photographs appearing in this book are of brand-name psychiatric drugs. In many cases, generic equivalents exist and will look different. While these photographs were accurate at the time of publication, from time to time drug manufacturers will change the appearance of the drugs they produce. Also, readers should bear in mind that the photographs in this book have been included for information only and that all issues relating to the appearance and use of these drugs should be discussed with a qualified health professional.

Acknowledgments

We would like to extend our gratitude to the following organizations for their important contributions to this book: Alzheimer's Association, American Anorexia Bulimia Association, American Psychiatric Association, American Psychological Association, American Sleep Disorders Association, Anxiety Disorders Association of America, Dean Foundation, Lithium Information Center, National Association of Anorexia Nervosa and Associated Disorders, National Depressive and Manic-Depressive Association, National Institute of Mental Health, and OC Foundation.

Special thanks go out to all of the kind and generous individuals who shared their personal experiences with us. We greatly appreciate your help, admire your strength, and wish you the best.

Last, but certainly not least, we would like to thank Peter Shure for introducing the two authors.

Contents

Introduction
How to Use
This Book

You've probably picked up this book for one of two reasons: you or someone you love is afflicted with a psychiatric disorder or you *suspect* that you or someone you love is afflicted with a psychiatric disorder. In either case, it may be somewhat comforting to know that you are not alone. At any given time, between 30 million and 45 million Americans—nearly one in five—suffer from a clearly diagnosable mental illness that interferes with everyday living. Consider these statistics:

- More than 9 million Americans suffer from depression each year. During any six-month period, an estimated 6.6 percent of women and 3.5 percent of men experience a depressive episode.
- Nearly 4 million people in the United States are trapped in the cycle of obsessive-compulsive disorder.

1

- One percent of teenage girls in this country develop anorexia, and up to 5 percent of college-age women are bulimic.
- Schizophrenia, the most baffling and debilitating of all mental illnesses, affects an estimated 2 million people in the United States each year.
- Twenty percent of the conditions for which we seek medical care are related to psychiatric disorders that interfere with our ability to live normal lives.
- Nearly one-fourth of the elderly who are labeled senile actually suffer from some form of mental illness that can be effectively treated.

Although most psychiatric disorders can be effectively treated or controlled, only one in five people with such problems seeks professional help. Many wrongly believe that their symptoms are their own fault or the result of personal weakness. They assume that if they try hard enough, they can overcome their problems on their own. In reality, however, many mental illnesses involve biological dysfunctions that require treatment by an experienced psychiatrist.

The fact that you're reading this book is a great sign. It means you've decided to take a first step in the right direction and help yourself or someone you love. We strongly suggest that you start out by reading the chapter entitled "Psychiatric Drug Therapy: A Primer." In it you'll find useful information about the warning signs of mental illness, drug therapy versus talk therapy, who practices drug therapy and psychotherapy, the various types of psychotherapy, how to find a psychiatrist, how a diagnosis is made, and what to expect during psychiatric drug therapy.

No doubt you've also picked up this book because you're interested in finding out more about the best-selling antidepressant in the country—Prozac. Since its release in the United States in 1988, more than 10 million people have taken Prozac for a variety of conditions such as depression, obsessive-compulsive disorder, bulimia, panic disorder, and attention deficit disorder, just to name a few. In only a handful of years, the drug has become so deeply ingrained in our culture that we wouldn't be surprised if nearly *everyone* in the United States knew at least one person who has taken it.

Prozac's rise to the top of the pharmaceutical market hasn't been without incident, however. Since early 1990, the drug has been linked to suicide and homicide as well as "personality transformation," prompting a barrage of questions from confused and concerned consumers. Is it safe for me to take Prozac? Is it going to make me commit suicide? Does it drive ordinary people to homicide? Will it make me more outgoing? Will it improve my social life? You'll find the answers to these questions and many more in the chapter entitled "Prozac: The Facts Behind the Fiction."

The remainder of the book is divided into two sections. The first section serves as a general reference guide to some of the most common psychiatric disorders: Alzheimer's disease, attention deficit disorder, depression, eating disorders, generalized anxiety disorder, manic depression, obsessive-compulsive disorder, panic disorder, phobias, schizophrenia, and sleep disorders. Each chapter contains up-to-date information about symptoms and treatment as well as answers to some of the most frequently asked questions about the disorder.

The second section serves as a general reference guide to nearly sixty of the most frequently prescribed psychiatric drugs in the United States. Each medication "profile" contains information about the use of the drug, side effects, special precautions, food and drug interactions, recommended dosage, overdosage, and pregnancy and lactation. The drugs are organized in alphabetical order according to their generic name. Prozac, for example, is listed as fluoxetine. If you don't know the generic name of the drug you want to look up, check the index. Both brand names and generic names are listed there.

As you read through the book, you'll notice that certain drugs are approved by the Food and Drug Administration (FDA) for the treatment of certain illnesses. Prozac is approved for depression and obsessive-compulsive disorder. Lithium is approved for manic depression. Xanax is approved for anxiety. Ritalin is approved for attention deficit disorder. What that means is the drug company has invested in the necessary clinical trials to demonstrate the effectiveness of the medication in treating a particular disorder. In the everyday world of mental health, however, psychiatrists routinely prescribe drugs for purposes that aren't approved by the FDA. That isn't bad medicine. In fact, it's good medicine.

If a body of clinical research strongly indicates that a drug has a nonapproved use, it's in the patient's best interest to try the drug. Several years before Prozac was approved for the treatment of obsessive-compulsive disorder, for example, psychiatrists across the country were prescribing it for the illness based upon existing scientific evidence. Another example is Tegretol. This anticonvulsant medication, used in the treatment of epilepsy, also happens to be a highly effective mood stabilizer and has emerged as an alternative to lithium in the treatment of manic depression. Yet, it will most likely never be approved by the FDA for that purpose because the FDA is not a proactive organization. It doesn't seek out drugs to approve. It's up to the manufacturer to submit an application for approval, and there are many reasons a manufacturer may choose not to go through the approval process. The company simply may not want to invest in the necessary clinical trials, for example.

One final note: This book is not intended as a substitute for a psychiatric evaluation. It is intended to provide you with a base of information about psychiatric disorders and psychiatric drugs. Only a psychiatrist can arrive at an accurate diagnosis and formulate an effective treatment plan. So if you or someone you love is suffering from a mental illness or you *suspect* that you or someone you love is suffering from a mental illness, take the next step. Seek professional help. It's not a sign of weakness. It's a sign of strength.

Psychiatric
Drug Therapy:
A Primer

We all have bad days. Days when we'd much rather stay in bed than face a stressful job, demanding family, or tough exam. Days when the frustrations of life take their toll on our patience or when preoccupation with the past or worries about the future chip away at our self-esteem. Times when we feel sad, anxious, angry, inadequate, or apathetic. Often, just talking about these feelings with friends or family members is enough to help us get through troubled times. But sometimes the problems don't go away, despite our best efforts to cope and the willingness of our loved ones to help. That's when it's time to seek professional help.

If you're not sure whether you or someone you care about needs to reach out for help, carefully consider the following warning signs of mental illness:

- *Distinct personality change.* Have family members, friends, or coworkers noticed that you don't seem to be yourself lately? Perhaps your spouse has mentioned that you seem distracted, or your best friend has pointed out that you don't seem interested in your usual recreational pursuits, or a colleague has commented that you seem on edge. Often, someone suffering from a psychiatric illness is the last to notice or admit that something is wrong. That's why it's important to carefully consider the observations and opinions of people you trust.

- *Difficulty performing daily activities.* Are your worries, fears, anxieties, or problems interfering with your ability to do your job or perform your usual tasks at home? A normal case of "the blues" usually doesn't prevent a person from fulfilling obligations at work, taking care of the children, or functioning in social situations. So if you're having trouble getting through your daily routine, it's a good idea to seek professional help.

- *Excessive anxieties.* Do you get depressed, anxious, or panicky for no obvious reason? If you've recently lost a loved one, it's perfectly normal to be depressed. If you have to give a speech in front of a large group of people, it's perfectly normal to be anxious. If you stumble upon a burglar in your home, it's perfectly normal to be panic-stricken. But if you find yourself depressed, anxious, or panicky for no apparent reason, you may be suffering from a psychiatric illness.

- *Prolonged periods of depression or anxiety.* Have your feelings of hopelessness or anxiousness lasted more than a few days? Normal, everyday worries and bad moods typically last only a day or two. So if you can't shake your worries or bad mood, particularly when family members and friends tell you that things aren't as bad as you think they are, you might need professional help.

- *Thoughts of suicide.* Have you thought that you would be better off dead? Any time that you seriously consider ending your life, you should pick up the phone and call 911 or another emergency number immediately or ask a family member or neighbor to drive you to the nearest hospital emergency room. Crisis intervention will prevent you from hurting yourself and help you find professional treatment for your depression.

- *Abuse of alcohol or drugs.* Do you drink or take drugs to help you get through the day? If you have a few drinks every night to forget about your problems, use someone else's tranquilizers to calm your nerves or help you fall asleep, or take illegal drugs to make yourself feel better, you should know that there are more effective remedies for anxiety, depression, and insomnia. A psychiatrist can point you in the right direction.

- *Bizarre or frightening behavior.* Do you find yourself coming up with grandiose schemes, such as taking over a major corporation or becoming a professional baseball player? Do you hear or see things that aren't really there? Many people walk to the beat of a different drummer in today's society, but there's a big difference between atypical behavior and psychotic behavior. If you or someone you know suffers from hallucinations or delusions, the best course of action is to seek psychiatric treatment immediately.

If you or someone you love displays one or more of these symptoms of mental illness, take that first step.

Get professional help. Remember, it's not a sign of weakness. It's a sign of strength.

Drug Therapy vs. "Talk" Therapy

If you've decided that you need professional help, the next step is to decide what type of professional help you need. Generally, there are two kinds of treatment for psychiatric illnesses—medication and psychotherapy (or "talk" therapy). For years, mental health professionals have hotly debated the pros and cons of these two treatment methods. On one side of the issue are psychiatrists who believe that all mental disorders result from abnormalities in the brain and should always be treated with drugs. To them, talk therapy is a waste of time. On the opposite side are psychotherapists who believe that psychiatric illnesses result from unresolved conflicts, adverse social conditions, negative experiences, or faulty thinking and should always be treated with talk therapy. To them, drugs simply cover up the symptoms of emotional problems.

Somewhere in the middle are those of us who believe that mental disorders are the product of a combination of biological, psychological, and social factors. As a result, we take a more holistic approach to treatment. We believe that a treatment plan should be tailored to meet the needs of the individual patient. Depending upon those needs, treatment may focus on drugs alone, psychotherapy alone, or a combination of the two. Since this book is about psychiatric drugs, much of the information contained in these pages is slanted toward drug therapy. However, it's important to note that we are not promoting medication as the only, or the best, solution to every psychiatric problem.

Types of Psychotherapy

You may be surprised to discover that there are literally hundreds of different approaches to psychotherapy. There are psychotherapies that focus on changing behaviors or thought patterns, psychotherapies that focus on exploring the effect of past relationships and experiences on present behaviors, psychotherapies that focus on treating troubled couples or families together, and psychotherapies that focus on tailoring procedures and methods to the needs of the individual . . . just to name a few. There are even psychotherapies that incorporate art, music, dance, and movement.

With such a dizzying variety of methods available today, it should be comforting to find out that most therapists practice one of, or a combination of, the following five approaches: psychodynamic, behavioral, cognitive, family, and supportive. Any of these approaches can be combined with drug therapy.

Psychodynamic therapy is based on the premise that unconscious, unresolved conflicts—fear of a critical mother, anger toward a distant father, feelings of jealousy toward a sibling—are at the root of emotional problems. To help solve emotional problems, psychodynamic therapists gradually coax these unresolved conflicts out into the open where they can be confronted and dealt with.

Behavioral therapy, in contrast, concentrates on altering specific, observable behaviors. If you have an irrational obsession with cleanliness and wash your hands dozens of times a day, for example, a behavioral therapist would focus on helping you reduce the number of times a day that you wash your hands instead of delving into the meaning behind the behavior and the unconscious conflicts that might trigger it. The assumption behind behavioral therapy is that emotional problems are learned responses and can therefore be unlearned.

Cognitive therapy, which is often combined with behavioral therapy, emphasizes the role that thoughts and patterns of thinking play in influencing behavior. The belief is that emotional problems result from negative, distorted, self-defeating thoughts, and that you can change the way you feel and behave by changing the way you think. Cognitive therapists work toward substituting distorted patterns of thinking with more realistic ones, thereby resolving the difficulties that those distorted patterns of thinking created.

Family therapy asserts that every couple and family has its own distinct culture complete with its own set of rules, roles, values, and problem-solving strategies, all of which influence the behavior of each member of the "unit." As a result, this approach involves all members of the unit—both partners in couples therapy and both parents and children in family therapy—not just the person experiencing "symptoms." The focus is not on changing individuals but on changing the way couples and families communicate and interact.

Supportive therapy, unlike the other four approaches mentioned, focuses on providing support rather than initiating emotional or behavioral change.

The emphasis is on bolstering your sense of self-esteem, supporting your strengths, and helping you deal with anyone or anything that threatens your ability to cope. Supportive therapy, for example, might be used to help you get through an acute depression or a psychotic episode, prevent relapses, keep your spirits up, and handle the demands of everyday living.

It's important to keep in mind that no one of these approaches is superior. In fact, the relationship between you and your therapist—how well you get along—is probably more important than his psychotherapy preferences.

Who Practices Psychotherapy and Drug Therapy

A wide variety of mental health professionals, including psychiatrists, psychologists, social workers, and psychiatric nurses, are skilled in psychotherapy.

Psychiatrists. Among these practitioners, only psychiatrists are licensed medical doctors. Psychiatrists attend four years of medical school, complete a one-year internship, and devote three more years to residency training in a hospital, clinic, or other medical center—just like internists, gynecologists, and pediatricians.

This medical background is important for several reasons. First, it uniquely qualifies psychiatrists to diagnose mental illnesses. Diagnosis is just as essential in dealing with mental disorders as it is in dealing with medical disorders. The decision to recommend drug therapy, psychotherapy, or a combination of both can only be reached after an accurate diagnosis has been made. Secondly, physical illnesses can sometimes trigger psychiatric illnesses, and psychiatrists are specially trained to recognize situations in which a medical disorder is masquerading as or worsening a mental disorder. Thirdly, psychiatrists are the only mental health professionals who are fully qualified to assess the benefits and side effects of psychiatric drugs. For these three reasons, it makes sense to see a psychiatrist at least once for a complete psychiatric evaluation. You'll find more detailed information on choosing the right psychiatrist on page 17.

Psychopharmacologists. Some psychiatrists are also psychopharmacologists, which simply means that they have special expertise in the use of medication to treat psychiatric illnesses. They treat psychiatric illnesses by prescribing various drugs at various doses, monitoring the blood levels of the drugs, adjusting the doses as needed, and meeting regularly with patients to talk about symptoms and side effects. Through this process, psychopharmacologists try to find the most effective combination of drugs . . . and often succeed. Some psychopharmacologists combine drug therapy with psychotherapy. Others prefer to focus on medication issues and assign the talk portion of the treatment plan to someone else, usually a nonmedical psychotherapist.

Psychotherapists. Unfortunately, there is no legal definition of a "psychotherapist" in most states. Anyone who has been told he is a "good listener" or has taken a psychology course at a community college can call himself a psychotherapist. For this reason, it's wise to choose a therapist with a degree in a mental health field, such as a psychiatrist, a psychologist with a Ph.D. or Psy.D., a social worker with an MSW, or a psychiatric nurse with an RN.

Psychologists. Like psychiatrists, psychologists are licensed mental health professionals who must meet state certification or licensing requirements to legally advertise themselves as psychologists. Typically, this requires a Ph.D. in clinical or counseling psychology or a related subspecialty, a one-year internship at a mental health facility, a specified number of hours of supervised clinical work, and a national licensing examination. The Psy.D., a relatively new degree, now also qualifies for licensing in many states. This course of study is geared more toward clinical practice and less toward research than traditional Ph.D. programs.

Social workers. In most states, social workers are also either certified or licensed. Generally, this procedure requires a master's degree in social work (which includes two years of course work and patient contact), two years of supervised postgraduate experience, and a qualifying statewide examination. Social workers who have expertise in the treatment of emotional and psychiatric problems are called clinical or psychiatric social workers.

Psychiatric nurses. All states either license or register nurses. Candidates must have a degree in nursing and pass a state examination. Psychiatric nurses receive additional, specialized training in mental health care through formal classroom instruction and/or hospital experience. Psychiatric clinical nurse specialists go on to earn a master's degree and receive supervised training in individual, group, and family psychotherapy.

Do You Need Two Therapists?

If your psychiatrist recommends both drug therapy and psychotherapy, you'll need to decide whether it's in your best interest to have your psychiatrist perform both functions or to separate the two functions. Each option has its advantages and disadvantages. Since the patient-therapist relationship can be emotionally turbulent, sometimes even adversarial, certain mental health experts feel that it's counterproductive to place a therapist in charge of dispensing medication. On the other hand, the argument for placing the same person in charge of both functions is that the close therapeutic relationship may enable the psychiatrist to understand how well the medication is or isn't working. The decision is usually yours to make.

In certain situations, however, the decision to combine or separate functions will be out of your hands. Some psychiatrists simply don't "do" psychotherapy and will automatically refer you to a colleague who specializes in that field. Others prefer to handle both the drug therapy and psychotherapy portions of the treatment plan. Your health insurance may also dictate the plan of action. Since psychiatrists are the highest-paid mental health professionals, your insurance provider may require a team treatment approach in which a psychiatrist oversees medication therapy and a lower-paid psychologist, social worker, or psychiatric nurse oversees psychotherapy.

A final note: If you're already working with a therapist whom you feel comfortable with, it's a good idea to continue working with him since he knows the specifics of your case. Rarely will a psychiatrist question the benefit of such an arrangement.

How to Find a Psychiatrist

If you have serious thoughts about committing suicide or feel you might hurt someone else, go directly to the nearest hospital emergency room. If you feel you can take the time to do some research in choosing a psychiatrist, however, take the following steps.

If you are already seeing a psychotherapist and think that medication might help you, discuss the matter with him and ask for a referral to a psychiatrist. This request shouldn't offend him. Good psychotherapists are open to biological interventions, just as good psychopharmacologists are open to psychological interventions. In fact, many psychotherapists have an ongoing relationship with a psychiatrist, a psychiatric group, or a mental health clinic. Your therapist's referral should include a detailed description of your symptoms and progress to date.

If you're not currently in therapy, start out with your family physician. Tell your doctor how you're feeling. He'll probably want to perform a complete physical examination to find out if any physical problems are contributing to your symptoms. If he recommends psychiatric treatment, ask for a referral to two or three psychiatrists who have experience in dealing with your specific problem or symptoms. (Feel free to specify age, gender, race, or religious background if that's important to you.) You should also request a copy of your medical records for the psychiatrist to examine.

Other good sources for referrals to psychiatrists include your local medical society, psychiatric society, community mental health center, and medical school. Medical and psychiatric societies can also tell you where the psychiatrists went to medical school and did their residency training and whether they're certified by the American Board of Psychiatry and Neurology. Family members and friends can be valuable resources as well. Personal chemistry is an important part of the therapeutic relationship, and the people who know you best are likely to have a strong sense of whom you'll feel comfortable with. Except for checking geographic location, the phone book is *not* the best referral source.

Check your health insurance policy to see if it will cover the treatment of psychiatric disorders. Many policies have arbitrary limits and may only cover 50 percent of the cost of a fixed number of visits per year. If your policy doesn't provide adequate coverage, talk to your employee benefits representative or insurance agent about improving it. Many employers offer several health care options, and you may be able to switch to a plan that allows for greater flexibility with psychiatric treatment.

Select two or three potential psychiatrists. Phone for information about appointment availability, location, and cost of the first visit. Then schedule an appointment. This initial consultation should last a minimum of one hour and may very well last an hour and a half or two hours, depending upon the policy of the particular psychiatrist.

The First Visit

During your visit, the psychiatrist will ask you many detailed questions in an attempt to form an accurate overall picture of your problem. Expect him to inquire about your current difficulties, prior difficulties, childhood, upbringing, family, education, job, social life, past and present living situations, habits, and general health. Because heredity is believed to play a role in the development of a number of psychiatric illnesses, he'll also ask if any blood relatives suffer from nervous or emotional disorders. In addition, he will want to know the date of your last complete physical examination, may ask to see your medical records, and may ask your permission to consult with your family physician. If you haven't had a recent physical, the psychiatrist will most likely perform one, send you to your own doctor, or refer you to another doctor.

Use this time to find out about the psychiatrist's fees, appointment flexibility, cancellation policy, and insurance form processing. It's also perfectly reasonable to ask him about his experience in prescribing psychiatric drugs, what percentage of his patients actually receive drugs, how frequently he uses drugs to treat patients with similar problems, if he specializes in treating specific types of psychiatric disorders, and his position on psychotherapy. It's important to point out that little, if any, treatment takes place during a first visit to a psychiatrist. The purpose of an initial consultation is for the psychiatrist to gather enough information about your problem to make a preliminary diagnosis. Once a diagnosis is made, treatment can begin.

After this initial visit, reflect on how you felt about the doctor. Did you feel safe? Did you feel comfortable talking about yourself and your problems? Did you feel understood? Did he seem genuinely interested in what you had to say and in what you were feeling? Did he welcome your questions? Did he talk in a way that you could understand? Is he a person you could trust? As a result of the meeting, do you feel better about your situation?

If your answer to any of these questions is no or even "maybe," or if the chemistry just didn't feel right to you, move on to the next psychiatrist on your list. When the chemistry *does* feel right, you've finished the first part of the job. The second part—working together with your psychiatrist to understand and overcome your problems—is about to begin.

How a Diagnosis Is Made

If a psychiatrist hasn't gathered enough information during your first visit to make a preliminary diagnosis, he'll schedule one or more follow-up sessions. After analyzing the details of your case, he'll then turn to the *Diagnostic and Statistical Manual of Mental Disorders (DSM)*. Since the early 1950s, psychiatrists have relied on the *DSM*, which is published by the American Psychiatric Association, to help diagnose mental illness. The latest edition, *DSM-IV,* is a carefully constructed index of psychiatric disorders grouped by categories and subcategories. It covers more than three hundred mental illnesses—from depression and manic depression to body dysmorphic disorder (a preoccupation with a defect in appearance) and trichotillomania (recurrent pulling out of one's own hair).

Each entry contains a general description of the condition followed by a listing of possible symptoms, which enables psychiatrists to identify specific psychiatric disorders with a high degree of accuracy, confidence, and objectivity. To be diagnosed as suffering from major depression, for example, you would have to display five or more of the following symptoms for two weeks or more:

- Depressed mood for most of the day, nearly every day.
- Markedly diminished interest or pleasure in all, or almost all, activities most of the day, nearly every day.
- Significant weight loss when not dieting, weight gain, or decrease or increase in appetite nearly every day.
- Insomnia or excessive sleepiness nearly every day.
- Observable restlessness or lethargy nearly every day.
- Fatigue or loss of energy nearly every day.
- Feelings of worthlessness or excessive inappropriate guilt nearly every day.
- Diminished ability to think or concentrate, or indecisiveness, nearly every day.
- Recurrent thoughts of death, recurrent thoughts of suicide without a specific plan, a suicide attempt, or a specific plan for committing suicide.

Although psychiatrists will use such descriptions to make diagnoses, there are few perfect fits in the diagnosis of *any* medical condition because symptoms may vary from person to person, both in their type and severity. For this reason, psychiatrists will observe a patient and his symptoms over time and sharpen the diagnosis based on any new information that this observation brings to light. People suffering from manic depression, for example, are often initially diagnosed as suffering from major depression since depressive episodes typically precede manic episodes. When the manic phase of the cycle strikes, then the diagnosis is changed from major depression to manic depression.

How Psychiatric Drugs Work

If, after studying the information gathered during the interview and consulting the *DSM,* a psychiatrist recommends drug treatment for your particular problem, be an informed consumer. Ask him how the drug works before swallowing a pill.

In a nutshell, nerve cells in the brain are separated by tiny spaces or "synapses." Chemicals called neurotransmitters send signals across these spaces, enabling the brain to do its job. Neurotransmitters all have specific shapes. Just as a key fits into an ignition switch, these chemicals fit into "receptors" on the surfaces of other cells. Researchers believe that mental illnesses can crop up if not enough neurotransmitters are in circulation, if they aren't able to make their way to the receptors, or if there are problems with the receptors. Psychiatric drugs are designed to correct specific imbalances.

It's equally important to ask the following questions before beginning drug therapy:

- What is the official American Psychiatric Association diagnosis of the condition?
- What nondrug therapies are most effective for this condition?
- Will nondrug therapy be used in conjunction with drug therapy?
- How likely is it that this drug will alleviate my symptoms or cure my problem?
- What are the possible side effects—both common and uncommon?
- Does my age, physical condition, or preexisting medical illness require any special precautions?
- Can the drug interact with any other drugs that I'm taking?

- How long does the drug take to work?
- How long should I continue to take it?
- Can I become addicted to it?
- Can I stop taking the drug at any time or does the dosage have to be reduced gradually?
- Will I experience withdrawal effects if I stop taking it?
- What else should I know about this drug?
- How much experience do you have in prescribing psychiatric drugs?

What to Expect During Drug Therapy

It's also essential to have a clear understanding of what psychiatric drug therapy is like before you swallow a pill. Unfortunately, prescribing psychiatric drugs isn't as easy as baking a cake. When you bake a cake, you know that if you measure out the ingredients properly, follow the directions carefully, and bake it for the specified amount of time, the finished product will come out of the oven looking similar to the picture in the cookbook. There is no cookbook for psychiatric drug therapy, however. Of course there are general guidelines and procedures, but psychiatrists have no foolproof "recipes" to follow.

Each one of the psychiatric drugs on the market can affect different people in different ways. One person may begin to notice an improvement in one week; another may have to wait three weeks for the drug to take effect. One person may respond well to a low dosage; another may require the maximum dosage to achieve the same results. One person may suffer from debilitating side effects; another may not experience any side effects. As a result, the right drug, or the right combination of drugs, is often found by trial and error.

So it's not a good idea to expect, as many people do, to walk out of a psychiatrist's office with a prescription, pick up the medication at the local pharmacy, feel better in a few weeks, and never look back. Such a scenario is the exception rather than the rule. However, it *does* take place on occasion. When twenty-three-year-old Debra decided to see a psychiatrist for her uncontrollable temper nearly two years ago, he prescribed fluoxetine (Prozac). Within a few weeks, she felt like a new person and experienced absolutely no side effects.

On the opposite end of the patient spectrum is forty-year-old Janet, who has been seeing psychiatrists on and off since she suffered from her first episode of major depression ten years ago. During the past decade, she has taken six different psychiatric drugs. Two of the medications left her feeling like a "noodle"—sedated and unmotivated. Another put her at risk for developing central nervous system damage. Another made her feel itchy on the inside. Yet another caused her to vomit without warning. Finally, two years ago, a new psychiatrist hit upon a drug that produced virtually no side effects for Janet. Needless to say, she was ecstatic.

Like Debra, Janet is an exception to the rule. It usually doesn't take ten years to find a drug that works well for a patient. However, it may take several months. During that time, you'll need to meet with your psychiatrist regularly, perhaps once a week, so that he can check for side effects and adverse reactions, monitor your progress, and perform any necessary tests. Once you're on a maintenance regimen, the visits may be reduced to once every few months. Certain drugs, however, require more frequent monitoring in the maintenance phase. Monoamine oxidase inhibitors, for example, are powerful antidepressants that have potentially serious side effects and can sometimes cause a patient to become "high." For this reason, many psychiatrists insist that people taking these drugs schedule an office visit once a month even after the episode of depression has passed.

Unfortunately, until your psychiatrist finds the most effective drug for you, there's little you can do except try to be patient and positive and have faith that relief is just around the corner. It's also worthwhile to keep in mind that short-term discomfort, inconvenience, and frustration is a relatively small price to pay for the long-term improvements you're likely to experience.

In the next chapter, you'll learn more about the drug that worked wonders for Debra. *Is* Prozac a wonder drug? Or is it just another product of media hype? You'll find the answers to these questions and many others by turning the page and reading "Prozac: The Facts Behind the Fiction."

2

Prozac:
The Facts Behind
the Fiction

Since its release in the United States in January of
1988, Prozac (known generically as fluoxetine hydrochloride) has been used by more than 10 million
people in the U.S.—more than 15 million worldwide—making it the most widely prescribed antidepressant in the world. Never before in the history of
the pharmaceutical industry has a drug attracted as
much attention, both positive and negative, as
Prozac. It has been hailed as a miracle drug and
denounced as a killer drug. It has been criticized and
praised for its ability to "transform personality."
Users have shared stories of success and recounted
tales of horror on television talk shows. Some 160
civil lawsuits have been filed against the manufacturer. The controversy continues today. That's why
we've dedicated an entire chapter to this drug.

Prozac first captured the interest of the media in

late 1989 and early 1990. *Newsweek* hailed it as a "breakthrough," and *New York* magazine labeled it a "wonder drug." Meanwhile, physicians couldn't write prescriptions fast enough as sales of the drug soared to $125 million in 1988, and $350 million in 1989. By 1990, Prozac had become the best-selling antidepressant in the world.

Then came the backlash. It started with a report in the February 1990 issue of the *American Journal of Psychiatry* documenting six cases of depressed patients who developed violent suicidal thoughts while taking Prozac. Several months later, a woman in New York filed a $150-million lawsuit against Eli Lilly and Company, the manufacturer of Prozac, charging that the antidepressant plunged her into an eighteen-month-long suicide spree during which she slashed herself more than 150 times. A week later, three families of victims murdered by a Louisville, Kentucky, man who shot twenty people and then killed himself while taking Prozac also sued the company for $50 million each.

In October of 1990, the Citizens Commission on Human Rights petitioned the Food and Drug Administration to remove Prozac from the market. (The group was founded by the Church of Scientology, which has been waging war on psychiatrists, psychiatric medications, and pharmaceutical companies since the late 1960s.) The flames were fanned yet again later that year when Prozac, along with several other psychiatric drugs, was discovered in the bloodstream of the man indicted for assassinating Rabbi Meir Kahane, founder of the Jewish Defense League. For months, newspapers and magazines sizzled with stories about the alleged link between Prozac and suicides and violent rampages. On television talk shows, "Prozac survivors" told sensational tales of selfmutiliation and assault. Support groups for people who claim they've had bad experiences with the drug also sprung up in a half dozen states.

Eventually, the news media moved on to a new controversy-in-the-making and Prozac managed to keep a relatively low profile until the 1993 release of *Listening to Prozac: A Psychiatrist Explores Antidepressant Drugs and the Remaking of the Self* by Peter D. Kramer. In this best-selling book, which quickly became a hot topic on the cocktail-party circuit, the author contends that Prozac has the ability to transform personality—to turn wallflowers into social butterflies, to give confidence to the chronically timid, to make the passive assertive. This appealing, yet unsettling, assertion prompted another flurry of articles and another set of questions: Is Prozac a personality pill? The psychiatric equivalent of a face-lift? A substitute for psychotherapy? What are the implications of chemically altering one's character? Are we in danger of turning into a homogeneous society populated by the eternally perky?

The comparatively unexciting fact behind the titillating fiction is that Prozac is neither a personality pill that erases individuality nor a killer drug that drives people to commit suicide or go on shooting sprees. It is simply a revolutionary new type of antidepressant that effectively treats certain, but not all, forms of depression as well as a number of other mental illnesses with surprisingly few side effects. That statement may not sell newspapers or magazines or attract television viewers—it's downright boring—but it happens to be the truth. In this chapter, you'll find many other truths about Prozac and discover, in the process, that truth isn't always stranger than fiction.

The Pre-Prozac Era

In order to fully appreciate why Prozac has become the best-selling antidepressant in the world, hitting $1.2 billion in sales in 1993, you need a crash course in basic brain chemistry. Nerve cells in the brain are separated by tiny spaces or "synapses." Chemicals called neurotransmitters send signals across these spaces, enabling the brain to do its job. Neurotransmitters all have specific shapes. Just as a key fits into an ignition switch, these chemicals fit into "receptors" on the surfaces of other cells.

Once a neurotransmitter has delivered its message, it is either broken down by enzymes and flushed out of the body or reabsorbed by the transmitting nerve cells and stored for later use. The latter process is called reuptake. Researchers believe that depression and a variety of other mental illnesses can crop up if not enough neurotransmitters are in circulation, if they aren't able to make their way to the receptors, or if there are problems with the receptors.

Before Prozac burst onto the scene, psychiatrists had two main classes of antidepressant drugs in their arsenal—tricyclic antidepressants (TCAs) and monoamine oxidase inhibitors (MAOIs). Both groups of medications, which have been around since the late 1950s, work by boosting the availability of various neurotransmitters and have proven to be highly effective in the treatment of depression. Unfortunately, it has also been proven that they can produce an array of unpleasant side effects.

TCAs can cause drowsiness, dizziness upon standing quickly, tremors, dry mouth, blurred vision, constipation, nausea, weight gain, increased sweating, increased sensitivity to sunlight, difficulty urinating, and difficulty reaching orgasm. MAOIs can lead to weight gain (sometimes as much as twenty pounds), trouble reaching orgasm, sleep disturbance, swelling around the ankles, dizziness, and low blood pressure. People taking MAOIs must also deal with the burden of following a strict diet since foods containing a naturally occurring substance called tyramine can interact with the drug and trigger a sudden, potentially life-threatening rise in blood pressure. Foods to forgo include aged cheeses, aged meats and fish, liver and liverwurst, broad beans, overripe bananas, pickled herring and pickled lox, beer, and wine. Certain prescription and over-the-counter drugs need to be avoided as well, including nasal decongestants, diet pills, and many cold, sinus, allergy, hay fever, and asthma medications. Unfortunately, these inconveniences often prompted people suffering from depression to drop out of drug therapy and attempt to live with the pain.

TCAs and MAOIs produce so many side effects because they affect several different neurotransmitters. TCAs block the reuptake of serotonin, norepinephrine, and dopamine in addition to blocking receptors for acetylcholine; MAOIs block the enzyme that breaks down serotonin, norepinephrine, and dopamine. Enter Prozac, the mother of a radically new class of antidepressants called selective serotonin reuptake inhibitors (SSRIs). As the term implies, Prozac blocks only the reabsorption of serotonin and not other neurotransmitters. Its most common side effects are similar to the side effects that you might experience as a result of drinking too much coffee—nervousness, stomach cramps, nausea, and diarrhea. Some people also get headaches, have trouble falling asleep, and experience delayed orgasm while on the drug.

Since Prozac is so much easier to tolerate than TCAs and MAOIs, physicians around the country have discovered that their depressive patients are much less likely to become drug-therapy dropouts. Prozac is also much easier for physicians to prescribe than the older antidepressants. Most patients start out by taking one full-strength, twenty-milligram capsule a day. TCAs and MAOIs, on the other hand, require users to undergo frequent blood tests and "work up" to a therapeutic dose over a period of weeks. This rather complex process, coupled with the potential side effects of TCAs and MAOIs, caused many physicians to prescribe antidepressants only for patients who were practically incapacitated.

Luckily, those days are gone. More depressed individuals are now receiving much-needed treatment thanks to the ease of use and easy-to-tolerate side effects of Prozac and other SSRIs such as sertraline (Zoloft) and paroxetine (Paxil). It's important to note, however, that SSRIs are no more effective than their antidepressant predecessors. Generally, 60 to 70 percent of people suffering from depression will improve after taking the first medication prescribed. The remaining 30 to 40 percent often need to be switched to a different dosage or a different class of drugs.

The Suicide Scare

As we mentioned earlier, the possibility that Prozac might make some people suicidal was first raised in a paper by doctors from Harvard Medical School published in the February 1990 issue of the *American Journal of Psychiatry*. The authors reported that six depressed patients developed, and became preoccupied with, violent suicidal thoughts several weeks after starting treatment with Prozac. Two tried, unsuccessfully, to kill themselves. The suicidal thinking ended when the drug was discontinued.

The media fed on this aspect of the article, largely sidestepping several critical points. Four of the six patients were taking other medications in addition to Prozac. Five suffered from other serious conditions such as alcoholism, bulimia, and manic depression. All six had long histories of "treatment-resistant" depression. And perhaps most significantly, all six had contemplated committing suicide or attempted it at some point in their lives. It's a fact that suicidal thoughts and/or actual attempts are one of the classic symptoms of depression. According to the National Institute of Mental Health, as many as 15 percent of people who suffer from severe depression eventually take their lives. So the Harvard report, although disturbing, is most certainly not a conviction of Prozac.

There are several possible explanations for the sudden suicidal tendencies that the six patients experienced. One theory, which has been supported by many psychiatrists, is that a small minority of people are so seriously depressed that they simply cannot summon up the energy to kill themselves even though they've considered suicide a viable alternative. After a few weeks of drug therapy, however, they gain the strength to act on their self-destructive impulses. This unfortunate phenomenon takes place because the energizing effects of *all* antidepressants, not just Prozac, kick in before the mood-elevating effects take hold. As a result, the risk for suicide ironically increases between the time drug therapy begins and the depression lifts—usually two to six weeks. Fortunately, careful monitoring by a psychiatrist can prevent people from harming themselves during this critical period.

While reviewing the Harvard case reports and subsequent case reports, a number of psychiatrists independently came up with another possible explanation. They noted that many of the patients who developed suicidal thoughts while taking Prozac also developed a sort of agitated restlessness, which they attribute to an unnerving condition called akathisia, a common reaction to certain antipsychotic drugs. People suffering from akathisia constantly feel like moving and are unable to sit still. This sensation of internal restlessness is often uncomfortable and aggravating enough to make people want to "jump out of their skin" or, conceivably, out of a building. Many psychiatrists are now convinced that akathisia, unwittingly brought on by Prozac, could very well trigger suicidal thoughts and/or behavior in a very small number of depressed individuals. The good news is that an experienced psychiatrist can identify symptoms of akathisia and either treat it or switch the patient to another medication.

Throughout the campaign against Prozac, the FDA has stood behind the drug. In 1991, it denied the petition by the Citizens Commission on Human Rights to take Prozac off the market. Several months later, an FDA advisory committee and an independent scientific advisory committee determined that Prozac and other antidepressants do not cause suicide or violent behavior. In fact, they declared, Prozac appeared to protect against violent behavior. Furthermore, scientific studies have shown that people taking Prozac are less suicidal than those taking a placebo or other antidepressants.

As far as the link between Prozac and homicide is concerned, a guilty verdict in the trial of a Michigan high school teacher in the summer of 1994 was the fifty-third criminal case in which the "Prozac defense" has failed. The teacher, who was convicted of first-degree murder in the shooting death of the school superintendent, claimed that the drug reduced his capacity to understand the nature of his actions. To date, the Prozac defense has been unsuccessful in every criminal case in which it has been used. Currently, some 160 civil lawsuits against Eli Lilly and Company are pending. A total of ninety-two have been dismissed so far.

The bottom line is that Prozac is not a killer drug. It, like any other drug, is imperfect. Unlike most other drugs, however, the strengths and weaknesses of Prozac have both been blown out of proportion.

A Personality Pill?

"Prozac [seems] to give confidence to the habitually timid, to make the sensitive brash, to lend the introvert the social skills of a salesman," writes Peter Kramer in *Listening to Prozac*. To illustrate his point, he tells the story of Tess, a wallflower with low self-esteem who blossomed into a social butterfly while taking Prozac. He also tells the story of Sam, an obsessional architect who mellowed out on the drug. Then there's Sally, an overly fearful woman who turned into a risk-taker. And there's Hillary, who was incapable of experiencing pleasure until she experienced Prozac. All of these individuals did much more than "get better" on the antidepressant; they were "transformed" by it.

That's all the media needed to read. Buoyed by a flurry of newspaper and magazine articles and talk show programs, the concept of personality transformation swept the country, and *Listening to Prozac* skyrocketed onto the best-seller list. To those looking for a quick fix, the possibility of becoming more confident, assertive, extroverted, energetic, optimistic, charming, and ultimately more attractive to the opposite sex simply by taking a pill every morning seemed wildly appealing. What many of those newspaper and magazine articles and talk show programs failed to mention, however, is that not all people on Prozac undergo such dramatic changes. "Some are unaffected by the medicine; some merely recover from depression, as they might on any antidepressant," Kramer himself writes on page 11. "[Only] a few, a substantial minority, are transformed."

Probably no more than 10 percent of people who respond well to Prozac experience anything that even remotely resembles a personality transformation. Some psychiatrists believe that these individuals are "hyperresponders," who react strongly not only to Prozac but to *all* antidepressants as well as stimulants. Others speculate that those who seem to be magically transformed suffer from a mild form of undiagnosed bipolar disorder, meaning that *any* antidepressant medication can easily push them into an overly elevated or "manic" mood.

The remaining 90 percent of people who respond well to Prozac simply recover, quietly and subtly, just as they might on a tricyclic antidepressant, monoamine oxidase inhibitor, or another selective serotonin reuptake inhibitor. Their depression lifts. Their symptoms disappear. Their eating and sleeping patterns return to normal. Their self-esteem rises a few notches. They feel more hopeful, upbeat, peppy, and alive. Often, these positive internal changes naturally lead to positive external changes such as a promotion at work, new hobbies and interests, improved personal relationships, or a revitalized social life.

These individuals are not so much transformed by Prozac as they are liberated from the shackles of their illness. No longer weighed down by depression, they are free to be who they really are. They don't take on a new personality; their original personality emerges. Many times, however, someone's original personality has been buried for so long that both he and his loved ones completely forget what it was like. Consequently, they may jump to the conclusion that the individual has undergone a major transformation like the kind described in *Listening to Prozac*. If this conclusion is correct, then *all* antidepressant drugs have the ability to transform personality.

The Multipurpose Medication

In December of 1987, the FDA approved Prozac for the treatment of depression. In March of 1994, it was approved for the treatment of obsessive-compulsive disorder. The following month, an advisory committee of the FDA voted unanimously in support of the use of Prozac in the treatment of bulimia. Currently, the advisory committee recommendation is being considered by the FDA.

Although Prozac has been officially approved for the treatment of only two mental illnesses, many psychiatrists successfully use it to treat a wide variety of conditions including attention deficit disorder, panic disorder, borderline personality disorder, phobias, substance abuse, premenstrual syndrome, obesity, kleptomania, and addictive gambling. Researchers believe that all of these conditions, and most likely

many more, are somehow related to the highly powerful neurotransmitter serotonin. This theory helps to
explain why Prozac and other SSRIs, which boost the
level of serotonin in the brain, appear to be useful in
alleviating the symptoms of these disorders.

Despite the fact that Prozac is prescribed for such a
broad spectrum of illnesses and has been used by
more than 10 million people in the United States
(more than 15 million worldwide), it is definitely not
a miracle drug. In fact, although it was originally
approved for the treatment of depression, it is not
effective for *all* types of depression. Many psychiatrists, for example, have found Prozac to be less
effective for melancholic depression and more effective for atypical depression. Melancholic depression
and atypical depression differ in several important
ways. People suffering from melancholic depression
are virtually incapable of being "cheered up." Individuals with atypical depression, on the other hand,
are capable of being cheered up by praise, attention,
personal accomplishments, good fortune, etc. Once
the source of the pleasure is removed, however, the
depression returns. In addition, individuals with
atypical depression tend to overeat and oversleep,
whereas sufferers of melancholic depression usually
lose weight and sleep poorly.

Prozac has also proven helpful in the treatment of
dysthymia. This mild form of depression often begins
in childhood or adolescence and lasts for years. Like a
low-grade infection, it prevents people from functioning at peak capacity, enjoying life, or feeling good.
Individuals with this disorder chronically feel "down
in the dumps" and "go through the motions" of life
with little enthusiasm or pleasure. Symptoms include
poor appetite or overeating, insomnia or hypersomnia (oversleeping), low energy or fatigue, low self-

esteem, poor concentration or difficulty making decisions, and feelings of hopelessness. Between 2 and 3 million people are estimated to suffer from dysthymia.

In order to qualify for an official diagnosis of major depression or dysthymia, according to the *Diagnostic and Statistical Manual of Mental Disorders,* an individual must display a specific number of symptoms over a specific period of time. A diagnosis of major depression requires the presence of five or more symptoms over a two-week period; a diagnosis of dysthymia requires the existence of two or more symptoms for at least two years. Many people meet these criteria, but many more don't. So what happens to people who display only three of the symptoms of major depression or only one symptom of dysthymia? They may be just as sick as those who exhibit the requisite number of symptoms, yet they aren't sick enough to merit an official diagnosis. The psychiatric community has a name for these individuals—the subclinically depressed.

Traditionally, people who suffered from chronic subclinical depression shuffled off to psychotherapy and spent months if not years talking about their low self-esteem, lethargy, lack of concentration, and overall misery. Unfortunately, most made little or no progress. Since Prozac came along, however, psychiatrists have discovered that the subclinically depressed respond much better to a combination of drug therapy and short-term psychotherapy than psychotherapy alone.

But why spend all that time and money in a therapist's office when you might be able to just take a trip to the pharmacy once a month? Contrary to popular belief, Prozac is not a replacement for psychotherapy. It is not a shortcut to healing. In fact, it can help people get more out of psychotherapy by enabling them to better focus on their problems. All Prozac does is improve an individual's mood and alleviate accompanying symptoms such as poor concentration and difficulties with eating and sleeping. It's then up to the individual to do the rest of the work on his own.

You'll find Prozac mentioned in the individual chapters on attention deficit disorder, depression, eating disorders, obsessive-compulsive disorder, panic disorder, and phobias. You'll also find a complete profile of the drug—including information about side effects, special precautions, food and drug interactions, recommended dosage, overdosage, and pregnancy and lactation—on pages 210–14. Armed with this information, you'll be able to make an informed decision in the event that your psychiatrist prescribes Prozac.

3

Overview
of Psychiatric
Disorders

Alzheimer's Disease

In 1907, a German physician by the name of Alois
Alzheimer identified a progressive disorder that
slowly kills nerve cells in the brain. Today, Alzheimer's disease (AD) is the fourth leading cause of
death in the United States. Only cancer, heart disease,
and strokes take more adult lives each year.

More than 4 million Americans are afflicted with
this degenerative disease. One in ten adults over the
age of sixty-five suffers from the illness; nearly half of
those over eighty-five have AD. Perhaps most alarm-
ing, it is increasingly cropping up in people who are in
their forties and fifties. Unless a cure or prevention is
discovered, more than 14 million Americans will be
afflicted with Alzheimer's disease by the middle of the
next century.

Sadly, the exact cause of Alzheimer's disease remains a mystery. One theory holds that nerve-cell death is related either to a decline in growth-promoting factors that maintain the functioning of brain cells or to a spontaneous increase in factors that are toxic to brain cells. Another theory links the illness to low levels of certain neurotransmitters. Researchers have discovered, for example, that people with AD have a deficiency of the neurotransmitter acetylcholine, which influences memory, thoughts, and other higher intellectual functions. Victims of the disease also have low levels of serotonin, the neurotransmitter that regulates aggression, mood, and sleep. Finally, scientists have found that some sufferers have a shortage of the neurotransmitter norepinephrine, which can contribute to anxiety, depression, excessive sleepiness, and difficulty in focusing attention.

Symptoms

In the beginning stages of Alzheimer's disease, sufferers develop almost imperceptible personality changes and short-term memory loss. They may seem more easily tired, upset, or anxious. They may become less spontaneous and avoid social interactions. They may repeatedly forget to turn off the stove or may grope for the right words in a conversation. Later in the course of the disorder, difficulties with abstract thinking and intellectual functioning develop. Victims may have trouble working with numbers, understanding written material, or organizing the day's activities. They also may become more agitated, irritable, and argumentative.

As the disease progresses and memory loss worsens,

affected individuals may ask the same questions over and over, not remember the date or season, be unable to describe where they live, and forget the names of longtime friends. Eventually, dementia sets in and sufferers begin to lose touch with reality. They may not be able to read, carry on a conversation, or recognize family and friends. They may become inattentive and erratic in mood, have long crying spells, grow suspicious and paranoid, need help dressing and bathing, lose bladder and bowel control, and become completely incapable of caring for themselves. Death, from pneumonia or another condition that develops in severely deteriorated states of health, usually follows.

This scenario represents the *general* range of symptoms for AD. Specific symptoms, along with the rate of decline, can vary considerably from person to person. Most people with the disorder can function at a reasonable level far into the course of the illness. From diagnosis to death, the average course of Alzheimer's disease is about six to eight years. However, it can range from three years to more than twenty years. Individuals who develop the disorder later in life often die from other illnesses, such as heart disease, before Alzheimer's reaches its final and most serious stage.

It's also important to keep in mind that none of the symptoms described above is unique to Alzheimer's disease. In fact, many conditions mimic AD, including side effects of medications, alcohol or drug abuse, decreased or increased thyroid levels, nutritional deficiencies, heart and lung problems, head injuries, and exposure to environmental pollutants such as lead, mercury, or carbon monoxide. Other serious illnesses, such as depression, diabetes, meningitis, multiple sclerosis, Parkinson's disease, and Huntington's disease, can also cause progressive dementia.

For this reason, the diagnosis of Alzheimer's disease is only made after all disorders that can bring on similar symptoms have systematically been ruled out. This requires a comprehensive clinical evaluation including at least three major components—a thorough medical examination, a neurological examination, and a psychiatric evaluation. Family physicians can often recommend the best way to go about getting the necessary examinations.

Treatment

Alzheimer's disease is not curable or reversible, but the symptoms may be alleviated and life made more bearable for both the sufferer and family. Tacrine hydrochloride (Cognex), which increases the availability of acetylcholine in the brain, is the only drug approved for Alzheimer's disease by the Food and Drug Administration. The medication is effective only for mild to moderate symptoms of the disease, however, and it only works for a small percentage of patients. Essentially, it sets back the clock of cognitive decline by about six months once the maximum dosage is reached. Users then continue to decline at the same rate. Side effects include nausea, vomiting, and diarrhea. A much more serious potential side effect is liver dysfunction, which must be monitored by weekly blood tests for the first several months of use.

Although tacrine is by no means a miracle drug, it represents an important first step in the treatment of

AD. It has demonstrated that symptoms of the disorder can indeed be reduced by boosting the availability of acetylcholine in the brain. As a result, an entire new area of research has opened up. Currently, several manufacturers are scrambling to develop drugs with similar mechanisms of action that are more effective and less toxic than tacrine. Like tacrine, however, they only slow mental decline. They don't reverse the course of the illness.

Other medications that often have a place in the management of Alzheimer's disease include antidepressants, which can increase appetite, improve sleep, and boost energy, and antipsychotics, which can keep paranoia, hallucinations, hostility, and agitation to a minimum.

Questions & Answers

Q. Is Alzheimer's disease hereditary?

A. That's a difficult question to answer. Most people who develop Alzheimer's disease don't have a family history of the disorder. Yet, in certain cases, it *does* appear to have a genetic link. This conflict has led some researchers to believe that there may be a number of different subtypes of Alzheimer's disease with different risk factors and causes.

Q. What tests are involved in the diagnosis of Alzheimer's disease?

A. A *definite* diagnosis of Alzheimer's disease can only be made when an individual's brain tissue is examined under a microscope and changes characteristic of AD are discovered. Since there is no highly effective treatment for the illness, this procedure is almost always performed after death. As a result, people suffering from symptoms of the disorder often need to undergo an extensive battery of tests to determine whether the culprit is a "mimicking" illness. The diagnostic checklist often includes blood and urine analysis, chest X rays, an electrocardiogram (EKG), a computerized axial tomography (CAT) scan, magnetic resonance imaging (MRI), and an electroencephalograph (EEG). Neuropsychological testing also plays an important role in the diagnosis of AD. Many tests now exist to measure very specific abilities, such as different types of memory (short-term, long-term, procedural), language, attention, abstract thought (concept formation, problem solving), and visual-spatial abilities (perception, orientation). Because the testing procedure is complex, some experts suggest that it be performed in an institution that specializes in spotting the disease.

Q. How long can people with Alzheimer's disease usually maintain a reasonable level of functioning?
A. It varies from person to person. Most people maintain the capacity for giving and receiving love, enjoying interpersonal relationships, and participating in a variety of activities far into the course of the disorder. A person with Alzheimer's disease may no longer be able to play chess, for example, but he may still be able to read a magazine. Playing the piano may not be possible, but singing along with family and friends may still be an option. Although driving may be out of the question, leisurely walks with family or friends may not be.

Q. Do all people with Alzheimer's disease end up in nursing homes?

A. Although at least half of the residents of nursing homes in this country have Alzheimer's disease or a related disorder, not every person with the illness must necessarily move to a nursing home. Many thousands of sufferers, particularly those in the early stages of the disease, are cared for by their families with the support of community services.

Q. How much does it cost to care for a person with AD?
A. The average cost of care in a nursing home is $36,000 a year. However, that figure can top $70,000 a year in some areas of the country. Home care costs an estimated $47,000 a year, $12,000 of which is typically paid for by insurance.

Q. What effect does Alzheimer's disease have on caregivers?
A. It can take a serious toll on caregivers. Caring for a loved one who is degenerating, both mentally and physically, can be an extremely painful and stressful experience. A study funded by the National Institute of Mental Health revealed that caregivers have increased rates of infectious illnesses and depression, as well as suppressed immune systems. Another study of caregivers found that 67 percent were angry. Researchers speculate that caregivers who hold in their anger may be at greater risk of cardiovascular disease.

Q. Where can family members go for support?
A. The Alzheimer's Association (800-272-3900), a nonprofit organization, operates some 220 local chapters around the country that run more than 2,000 family support groups, provide general information about the illness, help train home-care aides, and offer seminars on such practical topics as how to

make a home safe for people suffering from Alzheimer's disease. It's a valuable resource for anyone trying to learn more about or cope with the disorder.

Attention Deficit Disorder

They seem to be in a constant state of motion. They are extremely restless, have no patience, need constant stimulation, take unnerving risks, blurt out the first thing that comes to mind without considering the consequences, and jump from one task to another to another without finishing any of them.

It may sound like we're describing hyperactive kids, but we're actually describing adults. Little more than a decade ago, mental health professionals assumed that attention deficit disorder (ADD) was a childhood illness that faded with the onset of puberty. They were wrong. An estimated 50 to 70 percent of kids who have ADD continue to display symptoms as adults to a degree that seriously affects their lives. At least 4 million adult Americans, perhaps as many as 10 million, suffer from ADD.

Sadly, most are unaware that a very real neurological condition is at the root of their restlessness or that effective treatments are available. Most simply go through life convinced that they're lazy, ditzy, scatterbrained, self-centered, inconsiderate, rude, unmotivated, or immature. It's no wonder that many victims of ADD suffer from chronically low self-esteem, find it difficult to maintain relationships, perform poorly in school, drift from job to job, abuse alcohol or other drugs, get into accidents or trouble with the law, become depressed, or even commit suicide.

Many people with ADD escape diagnosis during childhood either because their symptoms are mild or because high intelligence helps them compensate for their difficulties. In kids, the disorder is often, but not always, marked by hyperactive behavior, including constantly fidgeting or squirming, having difficulty remaining seated, and talking excessively or out of turn. As they move into adolescence and adulthood, the hyperactivity often subsides, leaving behind distractibility, inattentiveness, impulsivity, and the inability to concentrate as the hallmark symptoms.

Since some ADD sufferers are hyperactive and others aren't, we've chosen to use the term *attention deficit disorder* in this book rather than *attention-deficit hyperactivity disorder,* which is the official term used in the *Diagnostic and Statistical Manual of Mental Disorders* published by the American Psychiatric Association.

Unfortunately, no one knows the exact cause of ADD. But a growing body of evidence points to a biological basis. Several studies have found that people with ADD have decreased blood flow and lower levels of electrical activity in the front lobes of the brain. Other research has shown that adults with ADD have lower rates of metabolism in areas of the brain that control attention, impulses, and motor activity. There also appears to be a genetic link. One expert estimates that 40 percent of kids suffering from ADD have a parent with the disorder, and 35 percent have a sibling with the condition. Pre- and postnatal injury (such as fetal alcohol syndrome, maternal smoking, and head trauma) may be involved in some cases. In others, exposure to toxic materials (such as lead or pesticides), allergies to food additives, or vitamin deficiencies may be responsible.

Regardless of the cause, proper treatment can help the vast majority of people afflicted with attention deficit disorder break the cycle of distraction and reclaim their lives.

Symptoms

At one time or another, we all have trouble concentrating, getting organized, meeting goals, dealing with frustration, keeping our temper in check, or following through on a boring project. In fact, for many people, feeling frazzled and distracted is a way of life in today's fast-paced society. How then do psychiatrists draw the line between an impetuous, energetic person who is feeling overwhelmed by the minutiae of life and someone who is suffering from a neurological disorder?

Most importantly, attention deficit disorder is not an adult-onset illness. A person doesn't wake up one day at the age of thirty and start displaying symptoms. The symptoms begin in childhood, typically before the age of seven, and continue into adulthood. Consequently, a woman who has found it difficult to concentrate and been easily distracted only since the birth of her child is not a likely candidate for a diagnosis of ADD. Someone who has had trouble concentrating and been easily sidetracked since elementary school, however, may very well have ADD.

To determine whether the condition dates back to

childhood, the psychiatrist must learn the history of the individual's life, including family history, pregnancy and birth history, medical history, developmental history, school history, job history, and interpersonal history. To accomplish this task, he may need to search school records and interview parents, siblings, and friends. Classic symptoms of ADD, outlined in the *Diagnostic and Statistical Manual of Mental Disorders,* that the psychiatrist or psychologist will look for include:

- Often doesn't pay close attention to details or makes careless mistakes in schoolwork, work, or other activities.
- Often has difficulty sustaining attention in tasks or play activities.
- Often does not seem to listen when spoken to directly.
- Often has difficulty following through on instructions and fails to finish schoolwork, chores, or duties in the workplace.
- Often has difficulty organizing tasks and activities.
- Often avoids, dislikes, or is reluctant to perform tasks that require sustained mental effort.
- Often loses things necessary for tasks or activities.
- Is often easily distracted.
- Is often forgetful in daily activities.
- Often fidgets with hands or feet or squirms in seat.
- Often leaves seat when it is inappropriate to do so.
- Often runs around or climbs excessively when it is inappropriate to do so. (In adolescents and adults, this symptom may be limited to subjective feelings of restlessness.)
- Often has difficulty playing or engaging in leisure activities quietly.

- Is often "on the go" or often acts as if "driven by a motor."
- Often talks excessively.
- Often blurts out answers to questions before they have been completed.
- Often has difficulty awaiting turn.
- Often interrupts or intrudes on others.

Before the psychiatrist determines that ADD is the culprit, he must rule out a host of other conditions that may accompany, mimic, or mask the disorder, including depression, manic depression, obsessive-compulsive disorder, post-traumatic stress disorder, hyperthyroidism or hypothyroidism, chronic fatigue syndrome, and substance abuse.

Treatment

There is no cure for ADD. As a result, the goal of treatment is to teach sufferers effective ways of coping with and compensating for the illness in order to minimize the negative effects of their symptoms. A combination of drug therapy and psychotherapy (including behavior modification) has proven to be the most effective treatment.

Drug therapy. In the late 1930s, a pediatrician discovered that stimulants had a calming effect on hyperactive children. Treating hyperactivity with stimulants may seem like a paradox, but it isn't. If, as researchers now suspect, most cases of ADD are caused by underactivity in an area of the brain that controls attention, concentration, and impulsivity, then stimulating this area of the brain should bring about a more balanced state. By the mid 1970s, the stimulant methylphenidate (Ritalin) had become the most prescribed medication for attention deficit disorder. It remains the drug of choice today.

Methylphenidate begins to work within thirty minutes to an hour after being taken. Its effects only last about three to four hours, however, so it must be taken several times a day. Most people take a dose at breakfast and another at lunch to make it through the school or work day. A sustained-release form of the drug, which can be taken once a day, is also available. Unfortunately, it isn't effective for everyone. The most common side effects of methylphenidate are insomnia, nausea, loss of appetite, and weight loss.

Alternatives to methylphenidate include dextroamphetamine (Dexedrine) and pemoline (Cylert). Like methylphenidate, dextroamphetamine must be taken several times a day since its effects only last about three to four hours. A once-a-day form of the drug is available as well, but it doesn't work for all ADD sufferers. Some psychiatrists prefer pemoline over both methylphenidate and dextroamphetamine because it produces fewer side effects and can be taken in a single dose. However, it doesn't work as quickly as other stimulants. Users may not notice an improvement for three or four weeks.

Other people respond better to antidepressants such as desipramine (Norpramin), imipramine (Tofranil), nortriptyline (Pamelor), and fluoxetine (Prozac). These drugs, like stimulants, work by increasing brain activity and promoting concentration. Specifically, they increase the amount of the neurotransmitters norepinephrine and serotonin.

Desipramine, imipramine, and nortriptyline belong to a class of drugs called tricyclic antidepressants. Side effects of these medications may include drowsiness, dizziness upon standing quickly, tremors, dry mouth, blurred vision, constipation, nausea, weight gain, increased sweating, increased sensitivity to sunlight, difficulty urinating, and difficulty reaching orgasm. Fortunately, these side effects usually fade after a few weeks.

Fluoxetine is a selective serotonin reuptake inhibitor, meaning that it blocks the reabsorption of serotonin by the transmitting nerve cell in the brain. One major advantage of fluoxetine is that its most common side effects are similar to the side effects that might be experienced as a result of drinking too much black coffee—nervousness, stomach cramps, nausea, and diarrhea. Some people also get headaches, have trouble falling asleep, and experience delayed orgasm while on the drug.

Nondrug therapy. Although medication is effective about 80 percent of the time, it alone is often not enough to transform a person who has spent all of his life in a perpetual state of distraction and disorganization. Behavior modification—learning how to impose order on everyday life—also is an essential part of treatment. Typical strategies include establishing a predictable schedule of activities, making lists of things to do, prioritizing tasks, using calendars and appointment books, setting deadlines, and assigning a location for possessions at work and at home. Surprisingly, these simple "nondrug" methods can work wonders for an ADD sufferer.

In addition to medication and behavior modification, many people with ADD also need individual psychotherapy to overcome lifelong problems with low self-esteem, negative thinking, depression, or anxiety. Another option is group psychotherapy, which gives ADD sufferers a chance to meet and interact with other people who have the disorder, talk about their experiences, share tips and coping strategies, receive emotional support, and feel connected.

Questions & Answers

Q. Are stimulants addictive?

A. They are definitely not addictive in the doses prescribed for ADD. Higher doses taken for long periods of time *are* addictive, however, and can cause severe side effects such as paranoia and delusions.

Q. Will I feel sedated on medication?

A. Absolutely not. If your psychiatrist prescribes the right medication and the right dosage, you'll feel less distracted, impulsive, frustrated, and anxious. In short, you'll feel "normal."

Q. What if the medication doesn't work?

A. If one medication doesn't work, another might. If the second doesn't work, a third might. If the third doesn't work, a combination of medications might. Because adult ADD is still a relatively new diagnosis, finding the right drug and the right dosage is often a trial-and-error proposition. The key is to keep trying, no matter how frustrated you feel.

Q. Will I have to take medication for the rest of my life?

A. Not necessarily. Some people need medication only until they master behavior-modification techniques. Others "mellow out" over time so that they can manage without medication. Still others *do* need to take medication for the rest of their lives. To determine which category you fall into, your psychiatrist will most likely discontinue drug therapy periodi-

54

cally—perhaps every four to six months—and monitor your response. You may find that you fare well without medication.

Q. How can I find a therapist to help me deal with ADD?
A. Your psychiatrist is a good place to start. If he isn't an expert on ADD, he may be able to recommend a colleague who is. Another option is to contact your local mental health association and find out whether there is an attention deficit support group in your area. Most support groups have a list of qualified professionals who regularly treat the disorder.

Q. How helpful are support groups?
A. For many people with ADD, self-help or support groups are a valuable source of emotional support, acceptance, encouragement, and friendship. In addition to referring participants to the best therapists in their area, support-group members share their personal experiences, learn coping skills, and distribute information about the disorder. Support groups for spouses of ADD sufferers are also springing up in a number of communities.

Depression

Everyone feels "down in the dumps" or gets a bad case of "the blues" from time to time. Not only are these emotions perfectly normal, they are an unavoidable part of the human experience. However, at some point a combination of the intensity and duration of these emotions suggests that the depression has ceased to be a temporary condition and has become a clinical state. Each year, more than 9 million Americans reach that point, according to the National Institute of Mental Health. Many are helped by the revolutionary antidepressant fluoxetine (Prozac). It has been used by more than 15 million people worldwide—more than 10 million in the United States alone—making it the most widely prescribed antidepressant in the world.

Clinical depression is much more than a bad case of the blues. It is a serious medical illness that affects an individual's moods, emotions, behavior, and thoughts. It affects his ability to concentrate and experience pleasure, the way he eats and sleeps, the way he feels about himself, the way he acts at home and on the job, and the way he views the world. No amount of "cheering up," exercise, vitamins, vacations, or prayer can make it go away. Neither can "keeping a stiff upper lip" or "toughing it out." Clinical depression is not a sign of personal weakness or lack of willpower. It is just as impossible to "snap out of" clinical depression as it is to "snap out of" pneumonia. Like pneumonia, clinical depression is an illness that requires proper treatment.

It also is an equal-opportunity illness. Depression strikes people of all ages, races, ethnic backgrounds, and socioeconomic levels. It affects the corporate executive, college professor, secretary, and auto mechanic alike. Nevertheless, some groups seem to be more affected than others. Women, for example, are twice as likely to suffer from depression as men. During any six-month period, approximately 6.6 percent of women and 3.5 percent of men will experience a depressive episode, according to the National Institute of Mental Health. Rates are also the highest for adults between the ages of twenty-five and forty-four.

As with hypertension, heart disease, diabetes, and cancer, scientists do not yet know the exact cause or causes of depression. What they *do* know is that it runs in families. Research has shown, for example, that if one identical twin suffers from depression or manic depression, the other twin has a 70 to 80 percent chance of being afflicted with the disorder as well.

Clinical investigations also suggest that depressed individuals have imbalances of the neurotransmitters serotonin and norepinephrine. Scientists believe that a decreased amount of serotonin may contribute to the sleep problems, irritability, and anxiety associated with depression, while a deficiency of norepinephrine may cause the fatigue and depressed mood associated with the illness.

Another area of vigorous research has focused on the hormone cortisol, which is produced by the body in response to stress, anger, or fear. In normal people, the level of cortisol in the bloodstream peaks in the morning and tapers off as the day progresses. In depressed people, however, cortisol peaks earlier in the morning and does not level off or taper off in the afternoon or evening.

A variety of other factors may also contribute to the onset of depression. It may be triggered, for example, by an acute or chronic physical illness (such as hypothyroidism or multiple sclerosis), certain prescription medications (such as steroids or antihypertensive drugs), certain recreational drugs (such as cocaine or amphetamines), or excessive alcohol consumption. Traumatic or stressful life events, such as a divorce, the death of a loved one, loss of a job, or move to a new city, may contribute to the development of the disorder as well. Many times, however, depressive episodes appear "out of the blue."

Symptoms

Symptoms of depression typically include:

- Persistent low, anxious, or "empty" feelings.
- Loss of interest and pleasure in activities previously enjoyed, including sex.
- Noticeable change of appetite, with either significant weight gain or weight loss not attributable to dieting.
- Noticeable change in sleeping patterns, such as troubled sleep, inability to sleep, early-morning awakening, or sleeping too much.
- Fatigue or loss of energy.
- Feelings of hopelessness or pessimism.
- Feelings of guilt, worthlessness, or helplessness.
- Inability to concentrate, make decisions, or remember details.
- Recurring thoughts of death or suicide, wishing to die, or attempting suicide.
- Aches and pains, constipation, or other physical ailments that cannot be explained.

Anyone who experiences five or more of these symptoms for at least two weeks, or whose everyday functioning has become impaired by these symptoms, may be suffering from *major depression*. This form of depression is one and a half to three times more common among first-degree biological relatives (children and siblings) of people with the disorder than among the general population. It also is twice as common in adolescent and adult women than in adolescent and adult men. Major depression can strike at any age, and its course is variable. Some people experience isolated episodes separated by many years of normal mood. Others suffer from clusters of episodes. Still others have more frequent episodes as they grow older.

Melancholic depression and *atypical depression* are two subtypes of major depression. They differ in several important ways. People suffering from melancholic depression are virtually incapable of being "cheered up." Nothing, not even winning the lottery, can lift their depressed mood. Individuals with atypical depression, on the other hand, *are* capable of being cheered up by praise, attention, personal accomplishments, good fortune, etc. Once the source of the pleasure is removed, however, the depression returns. In addition, individuals with atypical depression tend to overeat and oversleep, whereas sufferers of melancholic depression usually lose weight and sleep poorly. If left untreated, both melancholic and atypical depression can last for years.

Dysthymia is a less severe form of depression that often begins in childhood or adolescence and lasts for years. Like a low-grade infection, it prevents people from functioning at peak capacity, enjoying life, or feeling good. Individuals with this disorder chronically feel "down in the dumps" and "go through the motions" of life with little enthusiasm or pleasure. Symptoms include poor appetite or overeating, insomnia or hypersomnia (oversleeping), low energy or fatigue, low self-esteem, poor concentration or difficulty making decisions, and feelings of hopelessness. To be diagnosed with dysthymia, a person must suffer from two or more of these symptoms for at least two years. Sometimes people with dysthymia also experience superimposed major depressive episodes. Psychiatrists sometimes refer to this condition as "double depression."

Treatment

Although depression can be disabling, it is one of the most treatable mental illnesses. Between 80 and 90 percent of all depressed people—even those with the most severe symptoms—respond to treatment. The most effective treatment, a combination of medication and psychotherapy, helps to prevent or reduce both the length and severity of future depressive episodes.

The first step in the treatment is to undergo a complete medical examination to rule out the existence of another mental or physical illness since a number of medical disorders can sometimes produce depression. A person with symptoms of depression could be suffering from hypertension, hypothyroidism, or multiple sclerosis, for example. Or he could be reacting to substances such as barbiturates, benzodiazepines, or steroids. For this reason, a comprehensive evaluation by a qualified psychiatrist is vital to an accurate diagnosis. With this diagnosis in hand, the psychiatrist can then set out to design an appropriate treatment plan.

Drug therapy. Psychiatrists usually prescribe one of three types of medications to treat depression—tricyclic antidepressants (TCAs), monoamine oxidase inhibitors (MAOIs), or the newer "second-generation" antidepressants, fluoxetine (Prozac), sertraline (Zoloft), paroxetine (Paxil), trazodone (Desyrel), amoxapine (Asendin), bupropion (Wellbutrin), venlafaxine (Effexor), and nefazodone (Serzone). All antidepressants tend to bring mood, appetite, energy level, outlook, sleep patterns, and concentration back to normal.

Tricyclic antidepressants are often the drug of choice for the treatment of melancholic depression. In fact, 70 to 80 percent of people with melancholic depression respond to the first tricyclic prescribed. Imipramine (Tofranil), desipramine (Norpramin), and nortriptyline (Pamelor) are the most commonly prescribed TCAs. Others include amitriptyline (Elavil, Endep), doxepin (Adapin, Sinequan), protriptyline (Vivactil), and trimipramine (Surmontil).

Side effects may include drowsiness, dizziness upon standing quickly, tremors, dry mouth, blurred vision, constipation, nausea, weight gain, increased sweating, increased sensitivity to sunlight, difficulty urinating, and difficulty reaching orgasm. Fortunately, these side effects usually lessen after a few weeks.

Monoamine oxidase inhibitors such as phenelzine (Nardil) and tranylcypromine (Parnate) are often prescribed for individuals suffering from atypical depression or melancholic depression that has not responded to a tricyclic antidepressant. It is important to note, however, that the use of any MAOI requires patients to observe rigid dietary restrictions since foods containing the naturally occurring substance tyramine can interact with the drug and trigger a sudden, potentially life-threatening rise in blood pressure. Foods to avoid include aged cheeses, aged meats and fish, liver and liverwurst, broad beans, pickled herring and pickled lox, overripe bananas, beer, and wine. Certain prescription and over-the-counter drugs must be avoided as well, including nasal decongestants, diet pills, and many cold, sinus, allergy, hay fever, and asthma medications.

Many unpleasant side effects are also associated with MAOIs, including weight gain (sometimes as much as twenty pounds), trouble reaching orgasm, sleep disturbance, swelling around the ankles, dizziness, and low blood pressure. These side effects, as well as the side effects of tricyclic antidepressants, can often be minimized by beginning treatment with small daily doses that are gradually increased over the course of several days or weeks until an effective dosage is reached.

Of the half dozen second-generation antidepressants that have been introduced to the U.S. market since the 1980s, fluoxetine (Prozac) is by far the most widely prescribed. It belongs to a class of drugs called selective serotonin reuptake inhibitors (SSRIs) and is particularly effective in treating atypical depression and depression accompanied by panic attacks, obsessions and compulsions, or bulimia. One major advantage of fluoxetine is that its most common side effects are similar to the side effects that might be experienced as a result of drinking too much black coffee—nervousness, stomach cramps, nausea, and diarrhea. Some people also get headaches, have trouble falling asleep, and experience delayed orgasm while on the drug.

Two other SSRIs—sertraline and paroxetine—are effective as well. Like fluoxetine, they have minimal side effects. The most common include nausea, dizziness, sleepiness, insomnia, tremors, and increased sweating.

Trazodone and amoxapine also fall into the second-generation category. Amoxapine has the potential to cause a serious and at times permanent side effect called tardive dyskinesia. This neurological syndrome, which is associated with neuroleptic antipsychotic drugs, results in involuntary movements of the mouth, lips, and tongue such as tongue rolling, lip licking and smacking, chewing or sucking motions, pouting, and grimacing. Because this condition is so dreadful, and because so many other effective antidepressants are available, amoxapine is overlooked by many psychiatrists. Trazodone, on the other hand, can cause priapism, a potentially dangerous condition characterized by prolonged, painful erections. As a result, many psychiatrists avoid prescribing it for men.

Bupropion, another second-generation antidepressant, was introduced in 1986 for the treatment of depressed individuals who could not tolerate or did not respond to traditional antidepressant therapy. The manufacturer withdrew it from the market a short time later when several cases of seizures were reported in patients with the eating disorder bulimia. It was reintroduced in 1989 with the cautionary note that seizures occur in approximately four out of every one thousand patients. Nevertheless, many psychiatrists remain reluctant to prescribe the drug even though it does not produce many of the side effects associated with TCAs and MAOIs.

One of the newest second-generation antidepressants on the market, venlafaxine, is chemically unrelated to any of its predecessors. Like TCAs and MAOIs, it influences the neurotransmitters serotonin and norepinephrine, which play an important role in regulating mood. Unlike TCAs and MAOIs, however, it produces minimal side effects. The most common side effects reported in clinical trials were nausea, sleepiness, dry mouth, dizziness, constipation, nervousness, increased sweating, weakness, abnormal ejaculation, and anorexia. As a result, venlafaxine is likely to become a drug of choice for major depression in the coming years.

Nefazodone, which was approved by the FDA for the treatment of depression in December of 1994, also influences the neurotransmitters serotonin and norepinephrine. Its most common side effects include nausea, sleepiness, dry mouth, dizziness, light-headedness, constipation, blurred vision, confusion, and abnormal vision.

Many sufferers of depression can be treated on an outpatient basis. Individuals in the midst of a serious depressive episode, however, often need to be hospitalized so that they don't hurt themselves. Once symptoms are under control, maintenance therapy typically continues for six months to a year. The dose is then slowly and cautiously reduced until the drug is discontinued completely. Some people respond extremely well to treatment with antidepressants. They either remain symptom-free for life or for many years after drug therapy ends. Others don't fare as well. They suffer from frequent episodes and as a result need to remain on a maintenance dose for life.

Psychotherapy. For people suffering from mild depression, psychotherapy or "talk therapy" may be the only treatment needed. For the majority of depressed individuals, however, a combination of drug therapy and psychotherapy is far more effective.

Psychotherapy is beneficial in many ways. It can help sufferers of depression understand the illness, work through personal and emotional problems, improve their social functioning, and cope with stressful situations that could otherwise trigger another depressive episode. Two types of psychotherapy—cognitive therapy and interpersonal therapy—have proven to be particularly effective in treating depression.

Cognitive therapy emphasizes the role that thoughts and patterns of thinking play in influencing behavior. The belief is that emotional problems result from negative, distorted, self-defeating thoughts, and that you can change the way you feel and behave by changing the way you think. Cognitive therapists work toward substituting distorted patterns of thinking with more realistic ones, thereby resolving the difficulties that those distorted patterns of thinking created. Interpersonal therapy, in contrast, is based on the theory that troubled social and personal relationships can trigger depression. As a result, the interpersonal therapist concentrates on resolving the conflicts in the individual's relationships.

Both cognitive therapy and interpersonal therapy are short-term approaches to psychotherapy, typically taking place in ten to twenty sessions over a period of several months. For most people suffering from depression, this amount of time is sufficient. A small percentage, however, will need long-term psychotherapy.

Electroconvulsive therapy (ECT). In its early years, electroconvulsive or "shock" therapy earned a well-deserved bad reputation. Some psychiatrists used it haphazardly. Others used it as a threat to enforce the rules in mental institutions. When performed carelessly, it occasionally resulted in broken bones and other negative effects.

Fortunately, those days are long gone. Not only is ECT much safer today, it also is highly effective for treating people who are severely depressed, are at high risk for suicide, are severely malnourished, do not respond to antidepressant medication, or cannot take medication due to old age or medical problems. In these circumstances, ECT is often life-saving.

Under current ECT practices, the patient is briefly put to sleep with an intravenous anesthetic to ensure that he does not feel or remember the procedure. A muscle relaxant is then administered to reduce muscular response during treatment. Next, electrodes are placed on the head and a controlled pulse of electricity is applied. The treatment is usually repeated two or three times a week until the individual improves or it becomes obvious that further treatment will not be helpful. Most people respond within six to twelve sessions. Scientists believe that ECT works by affecting the same neurotransmitters that are affected by antidepressant medications.

Questions & Answers

Q. Is there a cure for depression?

A. Unfortunately, there is no cure for depression. Medications can *control* the condition the way insulin controls diabetes, but they don't *cure* it. Currently, the most effective treatment for depression is a combination of medication and psychotherapy. This two-pronged strategy helps to prevent or reduce both the length and severity of future depressive episodes.

Q. Can depression be prevented?

A. Scientists are trying to find ways to prevent or at least postpone the onset of a depressive episode, but we don't yet know whether this will be possible. However, we *do* know that proper treatment can either prevent future episodes or greatly reduce their intensity.

Q. If I have a genetic susceptibility to depression, does that mean it's just a matter of time before I develop a full-blown case?

A. No. All it means is that you may be vulnerable to depression when something upsetting takes place in your life, such as losing a loved one, ending a relationship, or leaving a job.

Q. Can depression lead to suicide?

A. Unfortunately, yes. If not properly treated, up to 15 percent of people hospitalized for severe clinical depression may eventually commit suicide due to the hopelessness, helplessness, and psychological pain associated with the illness. Although women attempt suicide more often than men do, men are two to three times more likely than women to actually kill themselves.

Q. How quickly do antidepressants work?

A. Antidepressants don't take effect immediately. It may take two to six weeks before you begin to notice an improvement. Hopefully, knowing about this delay will prevent you from becoming discouraged and "giving up" too soon. If the depression hasn't lifted after six weeks, your psychiatrist will most likely switch to a different medication.

Q. Will I have to take medication for the rest of my life?

A. That's a difficult question to answer. If the episodes of depression occur twice a year or more, if they're severe, or if they require you to be hospitalized, you may need to be on medication for the rest of your life. On the other hand, if the depressive episodes occur years apart or if you only experience one episode, you may only need to be on medication for six months to a year. Since the course of depression is hard to predict, however, it's important to discuss all the options with your psychiatrist before deciding to stop taking your medication.

Q. How helpful are depression support groups?

A. For many people with clinical depression, support groups are a valuable source of emotional support, acceptance, encouragement, and friendship. Support-group members share their experiences with the illness, learn coping skills, distribute information about new treatments, and refer participants to the best psychiatrists in their area. Support groups for family members and friends of depressed individuals are also available in many communities.

Eating Disorders

Dieting seems to be a way of life in the United States. At one time or another most of us have tried to lose five or ten pounds to fit into a favorite outfit, show off on the beach, impress a new love interest, or look better than our former classmates at a high school reunion. But for an estimated 8 million Americans, mostly girls and young women, what starts out as an innocent diet turns into a full-blown eating disorder.

Two of the most common eating disorders are *anorexia nervosa* and *bulimia nervosa*. People who suffer from either of these illnesses are overly involved with being thin, have an exaggerated fear of getting fat, and are obsessed with food. Yet, the symptoms are very different in nature. Anorexics literally starve themselves, eating a bare minimum of food and exercising excessively to burn the few calories that they do consume. Bulimics, on the other hand, eat enormous quantities of food in a short time (called bingeing) and then attempt to cancel out the calories either by vomiting, using a laxative, or taking a diuretic (called purging).

Over time, untreated eating disorders can lead to a host of serious and potentially fatal conditions. Anorexics, for example, often develop all the symptoms of starvation. They stop menstruating. They lose bone mass. They become constipated. Their breathing, pulse, and blood pressure fall. Their body temperature drops. Their joints swell and muscles waste away. Their hair and nails become dry and brittle. Their skin turns dry and yellow.

Most of the physical consequences of bulimia are actually side effects of bingeing and purging. Bingeing can result in abdominal pain and swelling, cramps, nausea, and inflammation of the pancreas. Vomiting can lead to tooth decay, a chronic sore throat, swollen salivary glands, weakness, fatigue, constipation, even heart failure. The abuse of laxatives and diuretics can cause dehydration, swelling of the fingers, mineral imbalances, and permanent kidney damage.

Several theories exist about the causes of eating disorders. Scientific research suggests that people who suffer from anorexia and bulimia have imbalances of neurotransmitters in the parts of the brain that control appetite, mood, and sleeping patterns. A low level of the neurotransmitter serotonin has been linked to bulimia, while a low level of the neurotransmitter norepinephrine has been associated with anorexia. Unfortunately, researchers don't yet know whether these biochemical imbalances *cause* eating disorders or are the *result* of the poor nutrition that characterizes the conditions.

Regardless, most psychiatrists believe that eating disorders can't be explained by biology alone. Psychological factors such as low self-esteem, they're convinced, play a major role in the development of anorexia and bulimia. An anorexic may feel, for example, that she is a failure in every aspect of her life except one—her ability to be thin. Similarly, a bulimic may view bingeing and purging as a means of controlling one aspect of her otherwise chaotic life.

The high value that society places on being thin, no doubt, also contributes to the development of eating disorders. Many people, even those who aren't necessarily overweight, simply can't attain the thin physique that has become so sought after in our culture. When a vulnerable individual tries, but fails, to meet societal standards, she may experience guilt, anxiety, fear, and loss of control. These emotional reactions, in turn, encourage her to diet again, and a potentially deadly cycle is set in motion.

Symptoms

The official diagnosis of anorexia includes the following four symptoms:

- Refusal to maintain a body weight that is minimally normal for her age and height (less than 85 percent of her expected weight).
- Intense fear of gaining weight or becoming fat, even though she is underweight.
- Disturbance in the way she experiences her body weight or shape (such as "feeling fat" even though she is emaciated), undue influence of body weight or shape on her self-evaluation, or denial of the seriousness of her currently low body weight.

- Absence of at least three consecutive menstrual cycles.

The official diagnosis of bulimia includes the following five symptoms:

- Recurrent episodes of binge eating (rapidly consuming a large amount of food in a short time).
- A feeling of lack of control during eating binges.
- Recurrent episodes of self-induced vomiting; misuse of laxatives, diuretics, enemas, or other medications; fasting; or excessive exercise in order to prevent weight gain.
- Bingeing and purging occur, on average, at least twice a week for three months.
- Undue influence of body shape and weight on her self-evaluation.

Treatment

Despite the fact that eating disorders are extremely complex and potentially life-threatening illnesses, most people suffering from them can be successfully treated if the condition is recognized early enough. Many individuals can be treated in a physician's office or clinic. However, some may need to be hospitalized if they're severely underweight, seriously depressed, or at high risk for suicide.

A psychiatrist's top priority in the treatment of anorexia or bulimia is to solve the physical problems associated with the illness. For anorexics, that means stopping weight loss. For bulimics, it means breaking the binge-and-purge cycle. Once this goal is reached, the focus of treatment shifts to a series of other hurdles such as correcting the person's distorted body image, boosting self-confidence and self-esteem, treating underlying depression, establishing normal eating habits, and preventing relapses. Generally, the total treatment plan for eating disorders includes a combination of drug therapy, individual, group, or family psychotherapy, cognitive-behavioral therapy, and nutritional counseling.

Drug therapy. Three types of antidepressant medications have proven to be effective in reducing the symptoms of bulimia—tricyclic antidepressants (TCAs), monoamine oxidase inhibitors (MAOIs), and selective serotonin reuptake inhibitors (SSRIs). In fact, research has shown that antidepressants can decrease the frequency of bingeing by as much as 70 percent.

Desipramine (Norpramin), imipramine (Tofranil), and amitriptyline (Elavil, Endep) are the most commonly prescribed TCAs. Side effects may include drowsiness, dizziness upon standing quickly, tremors, dry mouth, blurred vision, constipation, nausea, weight gain, increased sweating, increased sensitivity to sunlight, difficulty urinating, and difficulty reaching orgasm. Fortunately, these side effects usually lessen after a few weeks.

Phenelzine (Nardil), the most frequently used of the MAOIs, is also associated with several unpleasant side effects including weight gain (sometimes as much as twenty pounds), trouble reaching orgasm, sleep disturbance, swelling around the ankles, dizziness, and low blood pressure. In addition, the use of any MAOI requires patients to observe rigid dietary restrictions since foods containing the naturally occurring substance tyramine can interact with the drug and trigger a sudden, potentially life-threatening rise in blood pressure. Foods to avoid include aged cheeses, aged meats and fish, liver and liverwurst, broad beans, pickled herring and pickled lox, over-ripe bananas, beer, and wine. Certain prescription and over-the-counter drugs must be avoided as well, including nasal decongestants, diet pills, and many cold, sinus, allergy, hay fever, and asthma medications.

Of the SSRIs, fluoxetine (Prozac) has been studied the most. One major advantage of fluoxetine is that its most common side effects are similar to the side effects that might be experienced as a result of drinking too much black coffee—nervousness, stomach cramps, nausea, and diarrhea. Some people also get headaches, have trouble falling asleep, and experience delayed orgasm while on the drug.

Unfortunately, few controlled studies on the use of medications for anorexia have been conducted. Furthermore, those that *have* been conducted haven't produced conclusive results.

Psychotherapy. Various forms of psychotherapy can help anorexics and bulimics understand the emotions that trigger eating disorders, correct distorted body image, overcome the fear of gaining weight, improve self-confidence and self-esteem, change the obsessive-compulsive behaviors associated with food and eating, and adopt appropriate eating behaviors.

During cognitive-behavioral therapy, a form of individual psychotherapy, eating-disorder sufferers learn how to recognize the feelings that trigger abnormal eating behaviors and how to respond to those feelings in a new way. Group therapy enables people with anorexia and bulimia to help one another and themselves in an accepting, understanding, and supportive environment. Family therapy teaches loved ones about anorexia and bulimia, helps parents learn more effective parenting skills, enables family members to better understand their relationships with one another, and helps victims of eating disorders develop a strong sense of individuality.

The total treatment plan for anorexia or bulimia should also include a nutritional counseling component to help victims rebuild their physical health and establish healthy eating practices.

Questions & Answers

Q. Who gets eating disorders?

A. Of the 8 million Americans believed to suffer from eating disorders, an estimated 7 million are women. Research also indicates that 1 percent of teenage girls in the United States develop anorexia and up to 5 percent of college-age women are bulimic.

Q. Do parents cause eating disorders?

A. Problems with parents can *contribute* to the development and severity of an eating disorder, but they don't *cause* it.

Q. Does dieting cause eating disorders?

A. Not necessarily. While it's true that many anorexics and bulimics *did* diet before they became ill, most people who diet never develop an eating disorder.

Q. How does bulimia lead to tooth decay?

A. For starters, bulimics often binge on foods that are high in sugar, such as candy, cookies, cake, and ice cream. As a result, they tend to have a lot of cavities.

Secondly, the acid in vomitus eats away at tooth enamel. After a year or two of constant exposure to stomach acid, tooth enamel may wear off and teeth may begin to decay badly.

Q. Do laxatives really help to control weight?
A. No. By the time food enters the large intestine, the majority of its calories have already been absorbed. Over the course of a day, you'll lose *some* calories by taking laxatives, but not nearly enough to help you lose weight.

Generalized Anxiety Disorder

For many years, generalized anxiety disorder (GAD) and panic attacks were thrown together under the umbrella term *anxiety neurosis.* Recently, however, modern psychiatry has come to the conclusion that these two illnesses differ greatly and that generalized anxiety disorder is a legitimate condition worthy of its own diagnostic classification.

Unlike panic disorder, which is characterized by sudden attacks of intense and disabling anxiety, generalized anxiety disorder is a form of *chronic* anxiety. The GAD sufferer wakes up anxious and worried every morning and goes to bed anxious and worried every night. He worries excessively and unrealistically about nearly everything nearly all the time. He may worry about losing his job even though he just earned a major promotion. He may worry about developing a terminal illness even though he follows a healthy diet, exercises regularly, and has no family history of fatal diseases. He may even worry about minor matters such as grocery shopping, household chores, car repairs, or routine appointments.

No matter how hard a victim of GAD tries, he can't shake the feeling that "something bad" is going to happen. Often, it's just a matter of time before this twenty-four-hour state of worry begins to take a physical and psychological toll on him. He may feel restless and fatigued, experience headaches and heart palpitations, have trouble falling asleep, and drink excessive amounts of alcohol in an attempt to calm down. Despite the fact that these symptoms can create havoc in a person's life, many sufferers of the disorder don't seek professional help until they develop a full-blown depression or another subjectively serious mental disorder.

Symptoms

Generalized anxiety disorder is often difficult to diagnose because its symptoms are fairly vague and not easily observed. The most common symptoms are:

- Restlessness or feeling keyed up or on edge.
- Being easily fatigued.
- Difficulty concentrating or mind going blank.
- Irritability.
- Muscle tension, aches, or soreness.
- Difficulty falling asleep or staying asleep or restless sleep.

GAD sufferers may also experience such "garden variety" symptoms as trembling, twitching, heart palpitations, shortness of breath, sweaty palms, clammy skin, dry mouth, nausea or diarrhea, frequent urination, and trouble swallowing.

As a result, psychiatrists generally do not diagnose someone as having GAD unless the anxiety and worry is excessive and difficult to control, lasts for at least six months, is focused on a number of events or activities (such as family finances, a spouse's health, *and* household chores), is associated with three or more of the six major symptoms listed above, and significantly interferes with work performance, social activities, or personal relationships. A psychiatrist must also rule out the possibility that the person is suffering from another anxiety disorder with similar symptoms such as panic disorder, obsessive-compulsive disorder, post-traumatic stress disorder, or phobias.

Further complicating matters is the fact that a wide variety of prescription and over-the-counter medications can produce many of the symptoms of generalized anxiety disorder, including cold medicines, diet pills, allergy medications, antidepressants, sleeping pills, and blood pressure medications. Dozens of medical conditions, such as asthma, emphysema, encephalitis (an inflammation of the brain), heart disease, hypertension, hyperthyroidism (an overactive thyroid gland), and hypoglycemia (low blood sugar), can trigger anxiety symptoms as well. For these reasons, most psychiatrists recommend that their patients undergo a complete physical examination by a qualified physician before being treated for GAD.

Treatment

Once other possible causes have been ruled out and an accurate diagnosis has been made, nondrug treatments should be discussed and seriously considered before a prescription is written. One nondrug option that deserves special attention is aerobic exercise. Many researchers believe that regular, vigorous, aerobic exercise stimulates chemical changes in the body that reduce anxiety and increase a person's ability to tolerate discomfort and stress. For some GAD sufferers, a brisk thirty-minute walk every day may be the only treatment needed to relieve symptoms of anxiety.

Relaxation therapy is another useful tool in the management of anxiety. Massage, progressive muscle relaxation, meditation, yoga, and biofeedback are just a few of the many different types of relaxation strategies that often prove helpful in reducing anxiety, tension, and stress. Massage breaks down tension in muscles, sending a relaxation message back to the brain. Progressive muscle relaxation involves alternately tensing and relaxing various muscle groups in the body. People who meditate repeat a monotonous phrase or sound over and over as a method of inducing relaxation. Yoga is an ancient Hindu discipline that focuses on the control of the body and mind as a means of achieving tranquillity. Biofeedback, the most high-tech approach, involves hooking a person up to equipment that monitors heart rate, blood pressure, skin temperature, muscle tension, and brain waves. The subject is then taught to use mental techniques to lower heart rate or blood pressure, raise skin temperature, relax muscles, and even change brain waves.

Another noteworthy nondrug option is psychoanalysis or some other form of "insight-oriented" psychotherapy. This type of therapy is geared toward helping the individual uncover and resolve the emotional conflicts that may be at the root of his problems.

Drug therapy. If nondrug treatments fail, drug therapy is the next step. Throughout history, many substances have been used to calm people down, including alcohol, herbs, bromides, and more recently, barbiturates. Although barbiturates are effective antianxiety agents or tranquilizers, they are also highly sedating and addictive, often impair coordination, can trigger anger and depression, and can be lethal when combined with alcohol or taken in overdose. This harsh reality prompted scientists to search for safer compounds. Today, most drugs used to treat anxiety belong to a chemical group known as the *benzodiazepines*. In addition to being more effective than barbiturates, benzodiazepines have fewer side effects and are far less dangerous in overdose.

Benzodiazepines appear to work by enhancing the actions of the neurotransmitter gamma-aminobutyric acid, which reduces nerve-impulse transmissions and slows down certain brain activity. In the 1980s, researchers discovered that some brain cells have receptors that benzodiazepine molecules fit into as perfectly as a hand in a glove. This breakthrough led to the assumption that these manmade drugs somehow imitate chemicals made by the body that have a naturally tranquilizing effect.

All members of the benzodiazepine family are equally effective in treating GAD and begin to work fairly rapidly, usually within an hour or two. However, the rate at which they remain active in the body varies. Short-acting benzodiazepines, such as alprazolam (Xanax), lorazepam (Ativan), and oxazepam (Serax), are completely eliminated from the body within a few hours. Consequently, they are often reserved for situations in which the anxiety is likely to be short-lived. For a continuing effect, they must be taken several times throughout the day. Long-acting benzodiazepines, such as diazepam (Valium), chlordiazepoxide (Librium), clorazepate (Tranxene), clonazepam (Klonopin), and prazepam (Centrax), remain in the body for days. They can be taken in a single daily dose and are prescribed for people who are expected to need the drug for a long period of time.

The most prominent side effects of benzodiazepines are sleepiness, drowsiness, impaired coordination, and reduced alertness. Fortunately, these reactions usually become less pronounced after the first few weeks of treatment. Other side effects that may develop include muscular weakness, impaired memory, blurred vision, slurred speech, tremors, skin rash, excessive weight gain, and hypotension (low blood pressure).

Perhaps the most troublesome side effect is physical and psychological dependence, meaning that withdrawal symptoms may occur when benzodiazepine therapy is discontinued. Withdrawal symptoms can include irritability, restlessness, nervousness, insomnia, poor concentration, loss of appetite, headache, lack of coordination, perspiration, lack of energy, muscle aches, and sensitivity to light, sound, and touch. These adverse reactions can take place after being on benzodiazepines for just two to four weeks, which is why this class of drugs is used mainly for the short-term treatment of anxiety.

It is important to note, however, that the severity of the withdrawal symptoms depends upon several factors. Generally, the higher the dose of the benzodiaze-pine and the longer the person has been taking the benzodiazepine, the worse the withdrawal symptoms will be once the drug is stopped. Short-acting benzo-diazepines also tend to produce more severe with-drawal symptoms than long-acting benzodiazepines. In addition, withdrawal symptoms are likely to be more severe when the medication is abruptly discon-tinued. As a result, one of the best ways to minimize withdrawal symptoms is to reduce the dosage gradu-ally. This process could last anywhere from one week to several months depending upon the type of benzodiazepine (short-acting or long-acting), the dos-age, and the length of time the patient has been taking the drug.

A relatively new antianxiety medication called buspirone (BuSpar) has a dramatically lower risk of dependence than benzodiazepines, which means that GAD patients can take it for extended periods of time and stop taking it whenever they please without suffering from withdrawal symptoms. It also does not cause drowsiness or impair coordination or memory, but it can cause nervousness, light-headedness, in-somnia, upset stomach, nausea, diarrhea, and head-aches. The only major disadvantages of buspirone are that it must be taken several times a day and doesn't begin to take effect for several weeks, which may seem like several years to an extremely anxious person. As a result, people who need immediate relief are usually treated with benzodiazepines. Buspirone appears to work in part by enhancing the activity of the neuro-transmitter serotonin, which plays an important role in regulating activities such as sleep, mood, and aggression.

Questions & Answers

Q. Could my anxiety be caused by drinking too much coffee?

A. It depends upon how much coffee you drink. High doses of caffeine—the equivalent of two to four cups of strong coffee a day—can mimic many of the symptoms of anxiety, including headache, rapid breathing, nervousness, irritability, muscle twitching, hand tremors, and insomnia. Caffeine is also found in tea, cocoa, chocolate, and many cola drinks. So if you regularly consume large quantities of these products, it makes sense to decrease or eliminate your caffeine intake before seeking professional help. Many times even the most intense, prolonged cases of anxiety disappear when caffeine intake is drastically reduced.

Q. Does psychotherapy have a place in the treatment of GAD?

A. Definitely. Often, unresolved conflicts are at the root of chronic anxiety. As a result, an "insight-oriented" form of psychotherapy, such as psychoanalysis, often proves to be a valuable addition to the overall treatment program.

Q. If all benzodiazepines are equally effective in treating anxiety, what makes a psychiatrist choose one over another?

A. Psychiatrists often choose a benzodiazepine based upon its side effects. Lorazepam (Ativan), for example, has less effect on the liver than other benzodiazepines, so it's often prescribed for people who are taking ulcer medications, birth control pills, or other drugs that may affect liver function. Alprazolam

(Xanax), a high-potency benzodiazepine, is also effective in treating anxiety disorders that are complicated by depression.

Q. What will I feel like on benzodiazepines?
A. Like alcohol and virtually all other drugs, benzodiazepines affect different people in different ways. Typically, they produce a general state of well-being and make anxious people calmer, more relaxed, and less apprehensive. Since benzodiazepines make some people sleepy, however, your first dose should be small and taken at a time when you won't be driving or operating machinery.

Q. Can I become addicted to benzodiazepines?
A. The term *addiction* really doesn't apply to benzodiazepines. People who are addicted to a drug are completely consumed by it and will do anything to get their hands on it. People who take benzodiazepines definitely do *not* display that type of behavior. It's more accurate to say that people who take benzodiazepines can become dependent upon them and experience withdrawal symptoms when they stop taking them. Fortunately, the withdrawal symptoms only last a few weeks and aren't life-threatening. But they can make you feel quite uncomfortable—irritable, restless, nervous, shaky, lethargic. In rare instances, benzodiazepine withdrawal also causes convulsions.

Q. Can I die from an overdose of benzodiazepines?
A. While it's true that benzodiazepines are often used in suicide attempts, attempts made with benzodiazepines alone are rarely fatal. Unless you combine benzodiazepines with alcohol or other drugs, partic-

ularly barbiturates, you're not likely to die from an overdose. You're more likely to become very drowsy or stuporous or fall into a deep sleep. If you experience any of these symptoms, you should be taken to the nearest hospital emergency room immediately.

Q. Why can't I just take over-the-counter antihistamines to ease my anxiety?

A. Although antihistamines have some sedative properties and aren't habit-forming, they're not nearly as effective as benzodiazepines or buspirone in treating anxiety. Many people find that antihistamines cause so much drowsiness that they interfere with the routines of everyday life.

Manic Depression

All of us experience mood swings. Some days we're brimming with energy and enthusiasm. Other days we don't feel like getting out of bed in the morning. Not only is it perfectly normal to feel this way, it's an inescapable part of life. The more than 2 million Americans who suffer from manic depression, however, experience far more dramatic mood swings.

The illness is often called bipolar disorder because its victims cycle between two poles—from euphorically high or intensely irritable to hopelessly low—usually with periods of normal mood in between. When manic-depressives are up, they're *way* up.

When they're down, they're *way* down. During a manic phase, they might talk for hours without missing a beat, function on little or no sleep for days, start dozens of projects, and spend money lavishly. During a depressive phase, they might feel helpless and worthless, cry for no apparent reason, lose interest in all activities, and try to commit suicide. The difference between the two phases is that pronounced.

Manic depression also is an illness with many faces. Most people are plagued by repeated depressions and only an occasional episode of mania. Less commonly, mania is the main symptom and depression occurs only infrequently. Symptoms of mania and depression can even be mixed together in a single episode of bipolar disorder. The length of this up-and-down cycle also varies from person to person. Some individuals may experience a manic or depressive episode every few years. Others may be "rapid cyclers" and experience mood swings every few months, weeks, days, or even hours. Unfortunately, it is the rare individual who suffers from only one or two episodes in a lifetime.

Unlike depression, which can strike at any age, manic depression generally strikes in either adolescence or early adulthood. According to the latest scientific research, genetic factors play a significant role in determining who will develop it. Close relatives of people suffering from bipolar disorder are ten to twenty times more likely to develop either depression or manic-depressive illness than the general population. In fact, between 80 and 90 percent of people suffering from manic depression have relatives who suffer from some form of depression. If one parent has manic-depressive illness, a child has a 12 to 15 percent risk of developing a depressive disorder;

if both parents have manic depression, a child has a 25 percent chance of developing either a depressive disorder or a manic-depressive disorder.

Symptoms

Symptoms of the manic phase typically include:

- *An excessively good, euphoric, expansive, or irritable mood.* The person feels as if he is "on top of the world," and nothing—not even a horrifying event or tragedy—will stand in the way of his happiness. Often, however, this euphoria quickly turns into irritability or anger. (Irritability can also occur in the absence of euphoria.)
- *Unrealistic beliefs in one's abilities and powers.* Self-confidence may reach the point of "grandiose delusions." The individual may firmly believe, for example, that he has a special connection with God, that he is on a secret mission for the Federal Bureau of Investigation, or that he is going to become the next Wimbledon champion (even though he has never picked up a tennis racket). Or he may think that nothing—not even the laws of gravity—can prevent him from accomplishing a task. As a result, he may think he can step off a building or out of a moving car without being hurt.
- *Uncharacteristically poor judgment.* It is not uncommon for a manic-depressive to drive recklessly, spend money lavishly, make foolish business investments, become sexually promiscuous, or exhibit other questionable behaviors.
- *Hyperactivity.* Filled with boundless energy and enthusiasm, the person makes an excessive number

of plans or participates in an excessive number of activities. He may, for example, schedule several meetings, business appointments, lunches, and dinners in a single day, not realizing that there aren't enough hours in the day for all of them.

- *Flight of ideas.* The individual's thoughts race uncontrollably like a car without brakes careening down a mountain. When he talks, his words tumble out in a nonstop, although usually comprehensible, rush.
- *Decreased need for sleep.* Often, people suffering from mania go with little or no sleep for days without feeling tired.
- *Distractibility.* The person's attention is easily diverted to inconsequential or unimportant details.

If left untreated, the manic phase can last for months. As it wanes, the individual may experience a normal mood. But eventually the black cloud of depression begins to descend. Symptoms of the depressive phase typically include:

- Noticeable change of appetite, with either significant weight gain or weight loss not attributable to dieting.
- Noticeable change in sleeping patterns, such as troubled sleep, inability to sleep, early-morning awakening, or sleeping too much.
- Loss of interest and pleasure in activities previously enjoyed, including sex.
- Prolonged sadness or unexplained crying spells.
- Persistent feelings of worthlessness, hopelessness, or helplessness.
- Feelings of total indifference or guilt.
- Inability to concentrate, make decisions, or remember details.

- Recurring thoughts of death or suicide, wishing to die, or attempting suicide.
- Aches and pains, constipation, or other physical ailments that can't be explained.

These are the symptoms of *bipolar I* or "classic" manic-depressive illness. In another version of the disorder, *bipolar II,* the "highs" aren't as high. People trapped in the grip of bipolar II may plummet into deep depressions, but they don't skyrocket into psychotic manic episodes. Instead, they experience toned-down "hypomanic" periods during which they feel mildly euphoric, have lots of energy and self-confidence, and are highly productive, efficient, and creative. Unlike psychotic manic episodes, hypomanic episodes generally don't last long or prevent people from functioning on a day-to-day basis. In fact, they may even improve a person's work or social life. Consequently, individuals suffering from bipolar II may not realize that they have a problem and, in turn, may not seek medical help until the debilitating depressive phase of the cycle rears its head.

Cyclothymia, another form of manic depression, is one notch below bipolar II in terms of severity. The recurring highs and lows that a cyclothyme deals with are relatively muted and don't last long at all (a few days or weeks at most), but they're often pronounced enough to wreak havoc on the individual's life. People plagued by this disorder, for example, may move from place to place; change jobs, friends, or sexual partners frequently; start projects and never finish them; pick up hobbies or interests and suddenly stop pursuing them; or go on wild spending sprees.

Because manic-depressive illness has so many faces and courses, it is often not recognized by the individual, relatives, or friends and is often misdiagnosed by physicians. Further complicating matters is the fact that, in its early stages, bipolar disorder may masquerade as a problem other than mental illness. It may, for example, appear to be poor school or work performance or even substance abuse since many manic-depressives use alcohol or drugs to take the edge off their mania. Sadly, bipolar disorder tends to worsen when left untreated.

Treatment

Although manic-depressive illness can become disabling, it is also among the most treatable of the psychiatric illnesses. The first step in the journey is to undergo a complete medical evaluation to rule out the existence of another mental or physical illness since a number of medical disorders mimic manic depression. A person with symptoms of bipolar disorder could be reacting to substances such as amphetamines or steroids, for example. Or he could be suffering from multiple sclerosis or thyroid, liver, or kidney problems. For this reason, a comprehensive evaluation by a qualified psychiatrist is vital to an accurate diagnosis. (A general practitioner may not be familiar with all of the disorders that can masquerade as psychiatric illnesses.) With this diagnosis in hand, the psychiatrist can then set out to design an appropriate treatment plan.

The most frequently prescribed medication, lithium, successfully reduces the number, intensity, and duration of manic episodes for 70 percent of those who take it. (Twenty percent become completely free of symptoms.) It also wards off future episodes of depression, although somewhat less effectively than it prevents future episodes of mania. Those who respond best to the drug are individuals who have a family history of manic-depressive illness and who have periods of relatively normal mood between their manic and depressive phases.

Although lithium has been used to treat manic depression since the 1960s, nobody knows exactly how it works. Scientists believe that chemical imbalances in certain brain cells responsible for emotions and behavior are at the root of manic-depressive illness and that lithium corrects these imbalances.

Like all medications, lithium can have side effects and must be carefully monitored by a psychiatrist. Common side effects include fatigue, slurred speech, muscle weakness, nausea, stomach cramps, weight gain, increased urination, acne, swelling of the ankles and wrists, and impotence or reduction in sexual ability.

When an individual begins taking lithium, the physician measures the level of lithium in his blood at least once a week until a safe and effective level is reached. Achieving this "therapeutic" level is important because too little lithium isn't effective in stabilizing mood swings and too much can be toxic. Once the blood levels have stabilized, the test is repeated once a month for six months. After that, the lithium level is usually checked every three months for as long as the person is on the drug.

For those who don't respond to lithium, can't tolerate the side effects, or can't be managed on it alone, carbamazepine (Tegretol) and valproic acid (Depakene, Depakote) are effective alternatives. These anticonvulsant drugs, used in the treatment of epilepsy, may control manic-depressive illness by affecting the neurotransmitter gamma-aminobutyric acid. Unlike lithium, carbamazepine and valproic acid are mainly effective at keeping just the manic phase in check. They're often prescribed for "rapid cyclers" who experience four or more episodes of mania or depression a year. They're also well tolerated by most people. Common side effects include dizziness, drowsiness, nausea, and vomiting.

Questions & Answers

Q. Is there a cure for manic depression?

A. Unfortunately, there is no cure for manic depression. Medications like lithium *control* the condition the way insulin controls diabetes, but they don't *cure* it.

Q. Can manic depression be controlled without drugs?

A. Some psychiatric disorders can be treated successfully without drugs, but manic depression isn't one of them. If you're suffering from bipolar illness, you should be on medication.

Q. Will I have to take medication for the rest of my life?

A. If the episodes of mania or depression occur twice a year or more, if they're severe, or if they require you to be hospitalized, you'll probably need to be on medication for the rest of your life. If you stop taking your medication, the episodes of mania and depression will most likely return—maybe with even greater frequency and intensity. On the other hand, if the episodes of mania and depression occur years apart or if you only experience one episode, you may not need to be on medication continuously. Since the course of manic-depressive illness is hard to predict, however, it's important to discuss all the options with your psychiatrist before deciding to stop taking your medication.

Q. How quickly do the medications work?

A. The primary drugs used to treat bipolar disorder usually don't take effect immediately. It may take one to several weeks before you begin to notice an improvement. As a result, psychiatrists often prescribe additional medication to be used on a short-term basis until the primary medication kicks in. Hopefully, knowing about this delay will prevent you from becoming discouraged and giving up too soon.

Q. Will I need to be hospitalized when I start treatment?

A. If you're in the midst of a serious manic or depressive episode, you may not remember to take your medication properly or you may refuse treatment altogether. So you'll probably need to be admitted to a hospital, where medication can be administered regularly and you can be monitored closely. If you're in a "normal" mood, or your mood swings are moderate, you'll most likely be able to be treated on an outpatient basis.

Q. Will medication alone help me get my life back in order?

A. Medication helps to reduce or prevent future mood swings. It doesn't solve the personal problems that may have cropped up as a result of previous manic or depressive episodes. If manic depression has taken its toll on your relationships, family, career, and/or self-esteem, for example, you may benefit from psychotherapy or another form of counseling. Keep in mind, however, that it's impossible to "talk yourself out of" manic depression. Psychotherapy should always be viewed as a supplement to, not a replacement for, medication.

Obsessive-Compulsive Disorder

The executive who spends sixteen hours a day at the office . . . the woman whose house is so clean that it looks as though no one lives there . . . the new mother who checks on her baby a dozen times during the night . . . the teenager who tries on ten different outfits before going out on Saturday night. Are these people run-of-the-mill perfectionists, neat freaks, or worrywarts, or are they suffering from a mental illness? What's the difference between normal behavior and obsessive-compulsive behavior?

Essentially, there's a *big* difference between being neat and spending all day arranging the magazines on the coffee table, between practicing proper hygiene and washing your hands until they bleed, between being prudent and rechecking the door locks fifty times, between caring about your appearance and taking three hours to get dressed every morning, between being pious and reciting a prayer hundreds of times a day. People who act in an extreme way aren't run-of-the-mill perfectionists or neat freaks or worry-warts. They suffer from a surprisingly common disease called obsessive-compulsive disorder (OCD).

For many years, mental health professionals considered obsessive-compulsive disorder a rare illness because only a small number of their patients suffered from it. What they failed to realize is that many people afflicted with OCD do not seek treatment in an effort to keep their repetitive thoughts and behaviors a secret. However, a recent survey supported by the National Institute of Mental Health revealed that OCD affects nearly 4 million Americans a year, meaning it is more common than schizophrenia and other severe mental disorders.

Obsessive-compulsive disorder can strike at any age, but often begins in childhood. It affects people of all races and religions and in all economic brackets. It is also equally common in males and females. Although no one knows exactly what causes OCD, the fact that sufferers of the illness respond to specific medications suggests that it may be neurobiological in origin. In addition, more than 20 percent of people with OCD have family members who are also afflicted with the disorder. For these reasons, OCD is no longer attributed to attitudes learned in childhood—an inordinate emphasis on cleanliness, for example, or a belief that certain thoughts are dangerous. Instead, the search for causes now focuses on the interaction of neurobiological factors and environmental influences.

A growing body of evidence indicates that obsessive-compulsive disorder may involve abnormal metabolism in certain areas of the brain. Some researchers believe that overactivity in the front part of the brain leads to excessive concern with order, fastidiousness, meticulousness, *and* symptoms of OCD. Considerable evidence also points toward abnormalities in the functioning of a specific neurotransmitter called serotonin. Serotonin plays a key role in regulating activities such as sleep, mood, aggression, and repetitive behaviors.

Symptoms

OCD usually involves both obsessions and compulsions. Occasionally, someone afflicted with the disorder will experience obsessions only or compulsions only. Obsessions are intrusive, unwanted ideas, images, impulses, or worries that a person cannot stop thinking about. More often than not, the person experiencing the obsessions realizes that they are senseless and irrational, but cannot get them out of his mind. Extreme distress and anxiety is the result. Some of the most common obsessions include:

- *Contamination*—dwelling on becoming contaminated by shaking hands or drinking from a "strange" glass, for example.
- *Doubt*—such as wondering whether a door is unlocked, the gas stove is turned on, or the water is running.
- *Order*—an intense desire for symmetry and exactness.
- *Aggressive or horrific impulses*—a strong desire to hurt someone, for example, or shout out an obscenity in a place of worship.
- *Sexual imagery*—forbidden, perverse, or pornographic thoughts and images.

Compulsions are strong urges or drives to do something to reduce the distress and anxiety caused by obsessions. Usually, that "something" takes the form of a ritual. Someone tormented by doubts about having turned off the stove, for example, may try to ease his discomfort by checking it every few minutes. Someone with obsessions about becoming contaminated may wash his hands until they bleed. Someone plagued by pornographic thoughts may count to ten forward and backward one hundred times for each thought.

Some of the most common compulsive rituals include:

- *Cleaning*—Some OCD sufferers spend hours cleaning themselves and their surroundings. They may shower for most of the day, scrub the paint off the walls, or brush their teeth until their gums bleed. This compulsion afflicts more women than men.

- *Repeating*—Others with the disorder repeat behaviors, such as putting clothing on and then taking it off, saying the name of a loved one over and over, walking back and forth through a doorway, or touching certain objects.

- *Completing*—People who have this compulsion perform a series of complicated steps in an exact order. If the order is disrupted for some reason, they repeat the steps until the ritual is completed perfectly. A person may enter his home a certain way, for instance, taking four steps forward, two steps back, and humming one refrain of "God Bless America."

- *Checking*—The OCD sufferer's fear of harming himself or others develops into a ritual of checking.

He may repeatedly check the routes he drives to be sure he hasn't hit a pedestrian, or he may repeatedly check the front door to be sure it's locked. Men are more likely to be checkers than women.

- *Being meticulous*—Some sufferers of the illness develop an overwhelming concern about the appearance of a room or the placement of objects. They may spend most of the day arranging and rearranging magazines on a table at the expense of getting dressed or eating. An office worker may spend the day aligning and realigning the pencils on his desk instead of doing his job.

- *Avoiding*—Compulsive avoiders stay away from the object of their anxiety and any other object that is even remotely related to it. A person may be so fearful of chocolate, for example, that he avoids not only the candy but also anything else that is brown, including shoes, potatoes, and people with brown hair.

- *Hoarding*—Hoarders constantly collect, count, and stack useless items—anything from scraps of food to newspapers—to the point that rooms are filled, doorways are blocked, and health hazards develop. Hoarding is one of the less common compulsions.

- *Slowness*—Also a rather uncommon compulsion, which strikes mostly men, this compulsion prompts suffers to perform certain tasks extremely slowly. Shaving or polishing a table may require hours of painstaking effort, for example. Interestingly, slowness usually affects only one routine task; all other common tasks can be completed normally.

Most adults with OCD recognize that their obsessive thoughts are senseless and that their compulsive behaviors are useless. But this knowledge alone is not sufficient to enable them to break free from the obsessive-compulsive cycle—no matter how hard or how often they try. Time-consuming rituals eventually fill the day, making it impossible to lead a normal life. An executive who must follow a rigid dressing routine, for example, is chronically late for work. A student who must repeat his mother's name three times before he types each word of a term paper can't complete the assignment on time. A parent who must read the labels on food containers five times to ensure they don't contain poison doesn't get dinner on the table.

When left untreated, OCD tends to last for years, even decades. The symptoms may become less severe from time to time or may be mild for long intervals, but generally OCD is a chronic disease.

Treatment

Many people who display symptoms of OCD do not seek treatment because their obsessions and compulsions do not disrupt their everyday lives. Twenty-five-year-old Marianne, for example, is preoccupied with even numbers. As a result, she cuts her food into an even number of pieces and takes an even number of steps to get from one place to another. Since these compulsive behaviors do not interfere with her ability to function at work or at home, she sees no reason to get professional help. She simply incorporates her "personality quirks" into her daily routine.

Generally, a person is not diagnosed as suffering

from OCD unless the obsessive and compulsive behaviors cause noticeable distress, occupy more than one hour a day, or significantly interfere with his normal routine, functioning at work, social activities, or relationships. Unfortunately, many people who display these telltale symptoms prefer to hide their problem rather than seek treatment. As a result, they do not receive professional help until years after the onset of the illness. By that time, their obsessive-compulsive habits may be deeply ingrained and difficult to change.

Fortunately, there are two highly effective treatments for OCD—drug therapy and behavior therapy. Drug therapy helps to decrease both obsessions and compulsions. Behavior therapy provides sufferers with a method for reducing the anxiety caused by obsessions, which in turn reduces or eliminates compulsive rituals. Currently, the most successful treatment for nearly all victims of the disorder is a combination of drug therapy and behavior therapy.

Drug therapy. Over the years, a wide variety of psychiatric drugs have been used to treat OCD, including tranquilizers, amphetamines, antipsychotic drugs, monoamine oxidase inhibitors (MAOIs), tricyclic antidepressants (TCAs) and selective serotonin reuptake inhibitors (SSRIs). A handful are now known to have specific anti-obsessive-compulsive properties.

The TCA clomipramine (Anafranil) is the best studied of the anti-obsessive-compulsive drugs. It has a powerful effect on the neurotransmitter serotonin. Clomipramine increases the level of serotonin in the brain by delaying the recapture of the neurotransmitter. Its side effects may include drowsiness, dizziness upon standing quickly, tremors, dry mouth, blurred vision, constipation, nausea, weight gain, increased sweating, increased sensitivity to sunlight, difficulty urinating, and difficulty reaching orgasm.

Fluoxetine (Prozac), which also inhibits the reuptake of serotonin, has fewer side effects. In fact, the most common side effects of this SSRI are similar to the side effects that might be experienced as a result of drinking too much black coffee—nervousness, stomach cramps, nausea, and diarrhea. Some people also get headaches, have trouble falling asleep, and experience delayed orgasm while on the drug.

Two other selective serotonin reuptake inhibitors— sertraline (Zoloft) and paroxetine (Paxil)—have proven to be effective as well. Like fluoxetine, they have minimal side effects. The most common include nausea, dizziness, sleepiness, insomnia, tremors, and increased sweating. In December of 1994, a new drug called fluvoxamine (Luvox) was approved by the Food and Drug Administration for the treatment of OCD. Its most common side effects include sleepiness, insomnia, nervousness, tremors, nausea, vomiting, abnormal ejaculation, and sweating.

Psychotherapy. Of the several hundred types of psychotherapy being practiced in the U.S. today, a behavioral approach called exposure and response prevention has been found to be the most successful for people suffering from OCD. In this approach, a person is deliberately exposed to the situations that trigger his anxiety and is then prevented from carrying out the usual compulsive response. A compulsive hand washer, for example, may be urged to touch a dirty object and then denied the opportunity to wash for several hours.

Throughout behavior therapy, participants follow guidelines or a "contract" on which the psychiatrist and participants agree. The contract specifies whether the person is allowed to perform any part of his compulsive ritual and, if so, for how long and under what circumstances. A compulsive checker may be allowed to check door locks and gas stoves only once a day. A compulsive arranger may be permitted to reorganize the magazines on the coffee table for only ten minutes a day. When this technique is practiced over and over, the participant begins to learn that nothing bad happens if the rituals are resisted. As a result, the rituals gradually disappear.

Questions & Answers

Q. Is there a cure for obsessive-compulsive disorder?
A. Unfortunately, there is no cure for obsessive-compulsive disorder. Drug therapy and behavior therapy can *control* the condition the way insulin controls diabetes, but they don't *cure* it.

Q. Are people with obsessive-compulsive disorder delusional?
A. No, not unless they suffer from a separate psychotic disorder. The compulsive behaviors may seem delusional, but the people performing them are not. In fact, OCD sufferers are usually very aware of the excessiveness or irrationality of their fears or behaviors, yet they're unable to control them. This self-awareness often creates a new fear—the fear that others will think they are weak or out of touch with reality.

Q. How effective is behavior therapy?
A. Between 60 and 90 percent of people suffering from obsessive-compulsive disorder benefit from behav-

ior therapy. Typically, symptoms are reduced by 50 to 80 percent. It's important to keep in mind, however, that behavior therapy requires a substantial commitment of time and effort. It also requires you to face the very things you've been avoiding as well as to brave possible short-term increases in anxiety. For these reasons, 25 percent of OCD sufferers refuse behavioral treatment.

Q. How effective is drug therapy?

A. Anti-obsessive-compulsive drugs are effective for 50 to 80 percent of people with OCD. The average reduction in obsessions and compulsions ranges from 30 to 70 percent. Some people become virtually symptom-free.

Q. How long does it take for the drugs to take effect?

A. Unfortunately, the drugs don't take effect immediately. It may take two or more weeks before you begin to notice an improvement. Side effects, on the other hand, begin and usually are at their worst when drug therapy starts. Hopefully, knowing about these realities before you begin taking the medication will prevent you from becoming discouraged and giving up too soon.

Q. What happens when drug therapy is discontinued?

A. That depends on another factor. The bad news is that most people who haven't been treated with behavior therapy relapse rapidly. The good news is that people who *have* been treated with behavior therapy often maintain the improvements they've made.

Panic Disorder

Michael thought he was dying. While walking through an airport terminal, he was suddenly struck with an overwhelming and inexplicable sense of terror. For five endless minutes, his heart raced, he perspired profusely, his hands and feet went numb, and he couldn't catch his breath. The devastating attack left him in the fetal position on the terminal floor, sobbing and shaking uncontrollably. When the episode passed and he regained his composure, Michael wished that he *had* died during those five minutes. Then he wouldn't have to live in fear that the terror, without warning, would strike again.

Panic disorder is one of the most treatable mental illnesses. Tragically, it is also one of the mental illnesses most likely to be unrecognized, misdiagnosed, and incorrectly treated because it is so easily mistaken for other medical or psychiatric problems, such as heart disease, thyroid conditions, and respiratory ailments. This dilemma, coupled with the typical sufferer's tendency to keep his illness a secret, has made it difficult to gauge how widespread panic disorder is in the general population. However, a recent survey sponsored by the National Institute of Mental Health revealed that panic disorder affects an estimated 2.4 million Americans a year.

Little more than a decade ago, sufferers of panic disorder were dismissed as hypochondriacs or neurotics. Today, although the exact cause of the illness is still unknown, researchers believe that the ambush-like attacks are triggered by a biochemical abnormality. According to one theory, they take place when the brain's normal mechanism for reacting to a threat—the "fight or flight" response—becomes inappropriately aroused and an area of the brain called the locus coeruleus fires suddenly and unpredictably. Researchers have also found that panic disorder runs in families, indicating that genetics may play a leading role in determining who will develop the illness.

However, many people who have no family history of panic disorder are afflicted with it. First attacks are often triggered by a major life stress such as divorce or the loss of a loved one. Panic attacks may also strike for the first time after surgery, a serious accident, or childbirth. Other potential triggers include a high intake of caffeine, inhaling air with a high carbon-dioxide content, and using cocaine or other chemical stimulants, such as the drugs used to treat asthma.

Scientists also know that panic disorder typically strikes in young adulthood, although symptoms may crop up earlier or later in life. It affects people of all races and religions and in all economic brackets. Women, however, are twice as likely as men to suffer from it.

Symptoms

A panic attack is a brief episode of intense fear, lasting anywhere from several seconds to several minutes, that comes on suddenly without any apparent cause. The symptoms of such an attack may include:

- heart palpitations or racing or pounding heartbeat
- sweating
- trembling or shaking
- shortness of breath or sensations of being smothered

- choking sensations
- chest pain or discomfort
- nausea or stomach upset
- dizziness, light-headedness, or unsteadiness
- feelings of unreality or being detached from oneself
- fear of losing control or going insane
- fear of dying
- numbness or tingling sensations
- flushes or chills

People who suffer from repeated attacks and severe anxiety about experiencing another attack are diagnosed as having panic disorder. However, no two cases of panic disorder are exactly alike. The frequency and severity of the attacks often vary greatly from person to person. Some individuals may have attacks once a week for several consecutive months. Others may have daily attacks for a week and then remain symptom-free for weeks, months, or years.

Typically, a first panic attack appears to come "out of the blue" while someone is engaged in a routine, everyday activity such as driving a car or grocery shopping. Suddenly, the person is struck by a barrage of frightening symptoms. Convinced that he is having a heart attack or stroke, he rushes to the nearest hospital emergency room. Several hours later, after performing a battery of tests, the doctor on duty determines that the person is in no danger and sends him home with a prescription for rest and relaxation.

Buoyed by the doctor's assurance that "there's nothing to worry about," the panic-attack victim manages to convince himself that the crushing terror he experienced was an isolated incident and will never happen again. When another attack *does* take place, he tries to come up with an explanation and mistakenly attributes the cause of the attacks to the context in which they occurred. Someone who has had an attack while driving a car, for example, may believe that the act of driving or the road he was driving on somehow triggered the attack. As a result, he may refuse to get behind the wheel of a car again or to drive on that particular road again. Another sufferer may develop an irrational fear or phobia about shopping malls. Another victim may avoid elevators.

In addition to sidestepping places or situations that he fears will trigger a panic attack, the person begins to develop an intense apprehension about having another attack. This "fear of fear" is called anticipatory anxiety. The panic-disorder sufferer knows that an attack can strike anywhere, at any time, without warning, so he is always braced for it. Eventually, this pattern of phobic avoidance and anticipatory anxiety may progress to a more advanced stage in which the person becomes afraid of being in any place or situation that he might not be able to escape from in the event of an attack. This condition is called agoraphobia and affects about one-third of all people with panic disorder.

Typically, agoraphobics fear being in crowds, standing in line, being in shopping malls, riding in cars, or taking public transportation. Victims of the disorder often restrict themselves to a "comfort zone" that may encompass only home, work, and the immediate neighborhood. Venturing beyond the edges of this zone produces extreme anxiety. Sometimes a person with agoraphobia is unable to leave his home without a trusted companion or is unable to leave his home altogether. Needless to say, agoraphobia can be a seriously disabling condition. Sufferers of the illness may not be able to work and may rely heavily on friends and family members to take care of routine household errands such as going to the grocery store, bank, and post office.

Confined to a limited lifestyle that puts such a strain on relationships with family and friends, a panic-disorder sufferer is more likely to become depressed than the average person. In fact, recent studies have suggested that two out of three people with panic disorder experience depression at some point in their lifetime. Victims of the illness are also likely to turn to alcohol and illicit drugs such as cocaine and marijuana to alleviate the excruciating mental and physical symptoms of their condition. This form of "self-medication" is sadly ironic: alcohol and drugs tend to bring down mood and worsen anxiety, condemning the user to a downward spiral of anxiety, depression, and more panic. If left untreated, panic disorder can continue for years.

Treatment

It is not unusual for a panic-disorder sufferer to trudge from doctor to doctor in an effort to find out what is causing his symptoms. In fact, some victims visit more than a half dozen physicians and undergo extensive, costly, and unnecessary medical procedures before receiving appropriate treatment. The good news is that appropriate treatment effectively reduces or completely prevents panic attacks in 70 to 90 percent of people with the disorder. Early treatment can also help keep the illness from progressing to the later stages when agoraphobia develops.

The two most effective treatments for panic disorder are drug therapy and a type of psychotherapy called cognitive-behavioral therapy. In the past, mental health professionals have been divided on the issue of which approach works best. That debate continues to some extent today, but increasingly experts believe that a combination of medication and psychotherapy produces the best results—rapid relief from the crippling physical symptoms of panic attacks, a high degree of effectiveness, and a low relapse rate.

Drug therapy. Drug therapy is used both to prevent panic attacks and reduce their frequency and severity. The three groups of medications most often prescribed for panic disorder are tricyclic antidepressants (TCAs), high-potency benzodiazepines, and monoamine oxidase inhibitors (MAOIs). TCAs were the first drugs shown to be effective against the illness. Imipramine (Tofranil) is the tricyclic most commonly prescribed for panic disorder. Its side effects may include drowsiness, dizziness upon standing quickly, tremors, dry mouth, blurred vision, constipation, nausea, weight gain, increased sweating, increased sensitivity to sunlight, difficulty urinating, and difficulty reaching orgasm. Side effects usually lessen after a few weeks. It also usually takes several weeks for imipramine to work.

High-potency benzodiazepines such as alprazolam (Xanax), clonazepam (Klonopin), lorazepam (Ativan), and oxazepam (Serax) are also highly effective at heading off panic attacks. Unlike TCAs, they take effect quickly, are well tolerated by most people, and have relatively few side effects. The most prominent are sleepiness, drowsiness, impaired coordination, and reduced alertness. Fortunately, these reactions usually become less of a problem after the first few weeks of treatment. Other side effects that may develop include muscular weakness, impaired memory, blurred vision, slurred speech, tremors, skin rash, excessive weight gain, and hypotension (low blood pressure).

Perhaps the most troublesome side effect is physical and psychological dependence, meaning that withdrawal symptoms may occur when benzodiazepine therapy is discontinued. Withdrawal symptoms can include irritability, restlessness, nervousness, insomnia, poor concentration, loss of appetite, headache, lack of coordination, perspiration, lack of energy, muscle aches, and sensitivity to light, sound, and touch. The severity of the withdrawal symptoms depends upon several factors. Generally, the higher the dose of the benzodiazepine and the longer the person has been taking the benzodiazepine, the worse the withdrawal symptoms will be once the drug is stopped. Withdrawal symptoms are also likely to be more severe when the medication is abruptly discontinued. As a result, one of the best ways to minimize withdrawal symptoms is to reduce the dosage gradually.

Monoamine oxidase inhibitors are powerful antidepressants. Of the MAOIs that have been shown to be effective against panic disorder, phenelzine (Nardil) is used most frequently. It is important to note, however, that the use of any MAOI requires patients to observe rigid dietary restrictions since foods containing the naturally occurring substance tyramine can interact with the drug and trigger a sudden, potentially life-threatening rise in blood pressure. Foods to avoid include aged cheeses, aged meats and fish, liver and liverwurst, broad beans, pickled herring and pickled lox, overripe bananas, beer, and wine. Certain prescription and over-the-counter drugs must be avoided as well, including nasal decongestants, diet pills, and many cold, sinus, allergy, hay fever, and asthma medications.

Many unpleasant side effects are also associated with MAOIs, including weight gain (sometimes as much as twenty pounds), trouble reaching orgasm, sleep disturbance, swelling around the ankles, dizziness, and low blood pressure. These side effects, as well as the side effects of tricyclic antidepressants and benzodiazepines, can often be minimized by beginning treatment with small daily doses that are gradually increased over the course of several days or weeks until an effective dosage is reached. Treatment with all three classes of drugs generally lasts anywhere from six to twelve months. After that time, some patients remain panic-free for the rest of their lives. Others find that the attacks recur and opt to remain on medication for a longer time.

Newer antidepressants such as fluoxetine (Prozac), which belongs to a class of drugs called selective serotonin reuptake inhibitors, also appear to successfully counteract panic attacks. One major advantage of fluoxetine is that its most common side effects are similar to the side effects that might be experienced as a result of drinking too much black coffee—nervousness, stomach cramps, nausea, and diarrhea. Some people also get headaches, have trouble falling asleep, and experience delayed orgasm while on the drug.

Psychotherapy. As the term *cognitive-behavioral therapy* implies, this form of psychotherapy is a combination of cognitive therapy (which can modify or eliminate thought patterns that contribute to the symptoms of a panic attack) and behavioral therapy (which can help the individual change the way he responds to symptoms of a panic attack). Typically, a person undergoing cognitive-behavioral therapy meets with a therapist for one to three hours a week. During the cognitive portion of the session, the therapist tries to identify the thoughts and feelings that accompany the individual's attacks and in turn create a cycle of fear.

The cycle is believed to progress this way. First, the sufferer experiences a potentially worrisome sensation such as increased heart rate, shortness of breath, tightened chest muscles, or a queasy stomach. This sensation may be triggered by worry, unpleasant thoughts, minor illness, or even exercise. The person with panic disorder responds to the sensation by becoming anxious, which triggers more unpleasant sensations, heightening anxiety and eventually producing such catastrophic thoughts as "I'm having a heart attack." The result of this vicious cycle is a panic attack.

With the help of a skilled therapist, victims of panic disorder can often learn to recognize the earliest thoughts and feelings in this sequence and change their cognitive responses to them. Participants can learn, for example, to replace typical thoughts such as "I'm having a heart attack" with substitutes such as "It's only uneasiness. It will go away." Modifying thought patterns in this way helps to reduce anxiety and ward off a panic attack.

The behavioral portion of the therapy, which is usually multifaceted, may involve training in relaxation techniques. Learning to relax is another method of reducing the anxiety and stress that often set the stage for panic attacks. Breathing exercises are often included in behavioral therapy. Panic-disorder sufferers learn to control their breathing and avoid hyperventilation, a pattern of rapid, shallow breathing that can trigger or worsen attacks in some people.

Another important aspect of behavioral therapy is "interoceptive exposure" or exposure to internal sensations. During interoceptive exposure, the therapist encourages the participant to bring on some of the internal sensations associated with his panic attacks. The individual may, for example, exercise to increase his heart rate, breathe rapidly to trigger light-headedness, or spin around to cause dizziness. The therapist then teaches him to cope effectively with these sensations and replace alarmist thoughts such as "I'm going to die" with more appropriate ones such as "I'm just a little dizzy. I can handle it."

"In vivo exposure" or exposure to real-life situations is yet another essential component of behavioral therapy. During in vivo exposure, the therapist works with the participant to overcome the avoidance behaviors that are most seriously interfering with his life. The fear of driving may be most important to one person; the inability to go to the grocery store may be the biggest handicap for another. In all circumstances, the panic-disorder sufferer is encouraged to approach a feared situation gradually and stay with it despite rising levels of anxiety. After repeating this procedure a number of times, the individual begins to realize that his feelings, although terrifying, are not dangerous and do pass . . . and his small world begins to expand.

Questions & Answers

Q. Can psychiatric drugs "cure" panic disorder?

A. Drug therapy is used to *control* mental illnesses in much the same way that insulin controls diabetes. It doesn't *cure* them. In the case of panic disorder, however, drug therapy can be considered a cure in the sense that many sufferers remain panic-free after medication is discontinued. According to some mental health professionals, people who undergo a combination of drug therapy and cognitive-behavioral therapy are more likely to be "cured" than those who undergo either therapy alone.

Q. How long does cognitive-behavioral therapy usually last?

A. Cognitive-behavioral therapy requires a substantial commitment of time and effort to be effective in fending off panic attacks. Participants are generally in therapy for a minimum of eight to twelve weeks. Some people may need more time in treatment to learn and implement the skills. In addition to one-on-one contact with a therapist several times a week, this form of psychotherapy often involves doing a fair amount of "homework" between sessions.

Q. How helpful are panic-disorder support groups?

A. Many people consider self-help or support groups to be an essential part of their treatment program. Typically, a group of five to ten sufferers of the disorder meet weekly to share their experiences and offer encouragement. Family members are often invited to attend, and at times a therapist or other panic-disorder expert may be brought in to provide his insights. Group members are in charge of the sessions, which are almost always free of charge.

Q. Is traditional psychoanalysis effective in treating panic disorder?

A. Psychoanalysis focuses on uncovering the unresolved emotional conflicts that may be the cause of an individual's problems. This form of therapy alone is generally not considered effective in helping people overcome panic disorder or agoraphobia. It may help to relieve some of the stress that contributes to panic attacks, but it doesn't seem to prevent the attacks from taking place. However, if panic disorder is accompanied by other emotional problems, psychoanalysis or some other form of "insight-oriented" psychotherapy may be a helpful addition to the overall treatment program.

Q. How is agoraphobia treated?
A. Agoraphobia is usually treated in two steps. First, drug therapy is used to suppress the panic attacks. Then, a type of psychotherapy called behavioral desensitization is employed to help the sufferer venture beyond his comfort zone. Therapists typically begin by having the sufferer imagine a feared activity, such as walking to the mailbox, followed by talking about it with friends and family, and finally doing the activity in a series of small steps. Behavioral desensitization is a slow, gradual process.

Phobias

"My heart beats so fast that I feel like it's going to burst out of my chest. My throat tightens, and I have trouble breathing and swallowing. My hands start to sweat and shake. I get so dizzy that I have to hold on to something to keep myself from fainting or falling down." These words describe what a phobic person experiences when confronted with the object or situation that he fears.

Phobias are by far the most common of the anxiety disorders, affecting more than 20 million Americans a year, according to a recent survey sponsored by the National Institute of Mental Health. The term *phobia* refers to a group of psychological and physiological symptoms triggered by a feared object or situation. People can develop phobic reactions to virtually any object or situation—animals, elevators, heights, blood, flying, public speaking, even eating or drinking in public.

Symptoms

Phobias are persistent, irrational fears associated with certain objects, activities, or situations. The most common symptoms of a phobia include:

- Persistent, excessive, or unreasonable fear brought on by a specific object or situation such as dogs, insects, flying, heights, public speaking, or receiving an injection. Sometimes the mere *thought* of encountering the object or situation is enough to provoke intense fear.
- Immediate, uncontrollable anxiety when exposed to the feared object or situation. Symptoms of anxiety can include trembling, twitching, heart palpitations, shortness of breath, sweaty palms, clammy skin, dry mouth, nausea or diarrhea, and trouble swallowing.
- Recognition that the fear is excessive or unreasonable. Most people with phobias realize that their feelings are irrational yet are unable to control them.
- Avoidance of the feared object or situation. Some sufferers *are* able to confront the focus of their fear, but only with extreme anxiety or dread.

- Significant interference with a person's normal routine, job performance, social activities, or relationships. The fear of bungee jumping isn't considered a phobia because it doesn't affect daily living. An executive's fear of flying, on the other hand, may jeopardize his career.

Phobic disorders are generally divided into three categories—agoraphobia, specific phobias (formerly called simple phobias), and social phobias. *Agoraphobia,* which is more often than not an outcome of panic disorder, is discussed on page 106. A *specific phobia* is a fear of a specific object or situation. Virtually any object or situation can become the focus of this type of phobia. The most common specific phobia is a fear of animals, particularly dogs, snakes, insects, and mice. Other common specific phobias include fear of heights, closed spaces, flying, blood, crowds, germs, and thunder and lightning.

The level of anxiety that a phobic person experiences is usually proportionate to the degree of proximity to the feared object or situation. Someone who is afraid of cats, for example, will typically become more afraid as a cat approaches and less afraid as it moves away. The level of anxiety is also usually associated with the person's ability or inability to escape from a feared object or situation. Someone who is afraid of elevators, for example, will often become more distressed when an elevator is between floors and less distressed when the doors open.

Generally, sufferers of specific phobias do not fear the object or situation itself. What they fear is the potentially grim outcome of the encounter—being clawed by a cat, suffocating in an elevator stuck between floors, fainting at the sight of blood, crashing in an airplane, falling from a building, getting struck by lightning, etc.

Many phobic people "solve" their problem by simply avoiding the feared object or situation. Avoidance works particularly well when that object or situation rarely enters a person's life. If the focus of the phobia is a common object or situation, however, it may seriously hinder his ability to function on a daily basis. Someone who fears running water, for example, may not be able to shower, bathe, or brush his teeth. Specific phobias that have a negative impact on everyday living should be treated.

A *social phobia* is a fear of situations in which the person can be watched by others. In a sense, it is a form of "performance anxiety." But its symptoms go well beyond the normal nervousness that an entertainer may experience before an onstage appearance. Someone suffering from a social phobia may begin to sweat, blush, tremble, have heart palpitations, or even experience a full-blown panic attack when confronted with the feared situation.

The most common social phobia is the fear of public speaking. However, the focus of the phobia can be as ordinary an activity as making a telephone call, having a face-to-face conversation, answering a question in class, walking across a room, eating or drinking in public, or signing a check when the bank teller is watching. As in the case of specific phobias, victims of social phobias do not fear the situation itself. What they fear is the potentially humiliating consequences of the activity—sweating, stammering, or "freezing" during a speech or conversation, tripping and falling when walking across a room, trembling when eating, drinking, or writing in public, etc.

Also like sufferers of specific phobias, people with

social phobias tend to avoid situations in which they may be required to participate in the feared activity. They may, for instance, turn down dinner invitations or become withdrawn at school or on the job. The cost of such avoidance can be high—poor grades, missed career opportunities, broken relationships, social isolation, low self-esteem, depression, and alcoholism.

Treatment

The good news is that, with proper treatment, most phobia victims either improve greatly or completely overcome their fear. Furthermore, psychiatric research suggests that once a person successfully overcomes a phobia, he will remain symptom-free for years, if not for life.

Specific phobias. One of the most effective treatments for specific phobias is a type of behavioral therapy called exposure. The goal of exposure therapy is to force the participant to confront the focus of his fear without fleeing. *Systematic desensitization* and *flooding* are the two most common methods of exposure.

During systematic desensitization, the phobic person faces the feared object or situation in a series of steps. Therapists typically begin by teaching the individual various relaxation techniques to help keep the physical symptoms of his fear—heart palpitations, shortness of breath, trembling, twitching—under control. The next step is imagining the feared object or situation, followed by looking at pictures of it, and finally confronting the object of his phobia directly. Flooding, on the other hand, involves exposing the

phobic person to the feared object or situation immediately and encouraging him to remain until his
anxiety is significantly reduced.

Drugs are not typically used to treat specific phobias.

Social phobias. The treatment of choice for social
phobia is often a combination of behavioral therapy
and drug therapy. Effective medications include
selective serotonin reuptake inhibitors (SSRIs),
beta-blockers, and monoamine oxidase inhibitors
(MAOIs).

SSRIs such as fluoxetine (Prozac) increase the availability of the neurotransmitter serotonin in the brain.
Serotonin plays a key role in regulating activities such
as sleep, mood, and aggression.

One major advantage of fluoxetine is that its most
common side effects are similar to the side effects that
might be experienced as a result of drinking too much
black coffee—nervousness, stomach cramps, nausea,
and diarrhea. Some people also get headaches, have
trouble falling asleep, and experience delayed orgasm
while on the drug. Two other SSRIs—sertraline
(Zoloft) and paroxetine (Paxil)—appear to be effective as well. Like fluoxetine, they have minimal
side effects. The most common include nausea, dizziness, sleepiness, insomnia, tremors, and increased
sweating.

Beta-blockers, which are prescribed for high blood
pressure and angina, reduce the amount of stimulation by the nervous system to the heart and blood
vessels. As a result, they can be helpful in halting the
physiological symptoms of social phobia, such as
heart palpitations, tremors, sweating, and blushing.
Propranolol (Inderal) and atenolol (Tenormin) are the
beta-blockers most often used in the treatment of

social phobia. Both have negligible side effects in healthy individuals. They are more likely to produce side effects in people with asthma or other respiratory ailments, low blood pressure, heart conditions, diabetes, and hyperthyroidism.

Monoamine oxidase inhibitors such as phenelzine (Nardil) and tranylcypromine (Parnate) are powerful antidepressants. It is important to note, however, that the use of any MAOI requires patients to observe rigid dietary restrictions since foods containing the naturally occurring substance tyramine can interact with the drug and trigger a sudden, potentially life-threatening rise in blood pressure. Foods to avoid include aged cheeses, aged meats and fish, liver and liverwurst, broad beans, pickled herring and pickled lox, overripe bananas, wine, and beer. Certain prescription and over-the-counter drugs must be avoided as well, including nasal decongestants, diet pills, and many cold, sinus, allergy, hay fever, and asthma medications.

Many unpleasant side effects are also associated with MAOIs, including weight gain (sometimes as much as twenty pounds), trouble having an orgasm, sleep disturbance, swelling around the ankles, dizziness, and low blood pressure. For these reasons, MAOIs are generally used as a third line of treatment for social phobics who do not respond to SSRIs or beta-blockers.

Questions & Answers

Q. Who is the typical phobia sufferer?
A. Women are more likely than men to develop specific phobias. Social phobias, on the other hand, afflict

men and women relatively equally. This type of phobia generally develops after puberty and peaks after the age of thirty.

Q. Do specific phobias go away on their own?
A. Specific phobias typically develop during childhood and eventually disappear. Those that continue into adulthood, however, rarely go away without treatment.

Q. What causes social phobia?
A. No one knows for sure. Some psychiatrists believe that social phobia is the result of oversecretion of adrenaline or other stress hormones. Other mental health professionals insist that its roots are embedded in the subconscious. Still others contend that it stems from lack of assertiveness and inferior social skills.

Q. How common is depression among social phobics?
A. About one-third of people with social phobia also suffer from depression. Symptoms of depression include sadness, crying spells, feelings of worthlessness and hopelessness, loss of interest in activities previously enjoyed, noticeable changes in appetite and sleeping patterns, inability to concentrate, and thoughts of suicide.

Q. How common is alcoholism among people with social phobia?
A. Studies have indicated that 10 to 20 percent of social phobics are also alcoholics. Furthermore, research suggests that one-third of alcoholics have a history of panic disorder or social phobia. When alcoholism is associated with any anxiety disorder, it must be treated first.

Schizophrenia

Some hear voices and see things that aren't there. Some talk nonstop nonsense, randomly and incomprehensibly stringing words together. Others suffer from delusions, believing that they're in touch with aliens or being watched by the government. Still others appear emotionless and zombielike.

These are the many faces of schizophrenia, a term used to describe the most chronic, debilitating, and baffling of all mental illnesses, which affects an estimated 2 million people in the United States each year. Unlike most other psychiatric disorders, schizophrenia can alter virtually every aspect of a person's being—his thoughts, feelings, perceptions, sense of self, bodily coordination, social skills, interpersonal relationships, career, and ability to take care of himself.

An individual suffering from schizophrenia will typically cycle between two phases—an "active" phase during which he experiences psychotic symptoms such as hallucinations and delusions (also called "positive" symptoms), and a "remission" phase during which the psychotic symptoms subside. He may, however, continue to suffer from some deficits, such as difficulty with motivation or expressivity (also called "negative" symptoms), during remission.

Some people experience only one psychotic episode; others experience many but lead relatively normal lives during the interim periods. Most people with chronic schizophrenia do not fully regain normal functioning and usually require long-term treatment, including medication, to control the psychotic symptoms. For reasons no one understands, 10 to 30 percent of schizophrenics go into and maintain remission in the latter part of life—after the age of sixty.

Theories about the causes of the illness abound. It has long been known that schizophrenia runs in families, suggesting that genetics may play a role in determining who will develop it. Studies have shown that children with one parent suffering from schizophrenia have an 8 to 18 percent chance of developing the disorder. If both parents suffer from schizophrenia, the risk rises to between 15 and 50 percent. In comparison, the risk of schizophrenia in the general population is only 1 percent.

Research also has demonstrated that if one identical twin develops schizophrenia, the other twin has a 50 percent chance of developing it as well. This suggests, again, that genetics is an important determining factor. However, it is not the only one. Many researchers suspect that people inherit a susceptibility or vulnerability to schizophrenia, which can be triggered by environmental factors such as a viral infection that changes the body's chemistry, an unhappy or abusive childhood, a highly stressful event in adult life, or a combination of these and other factors.

In addition, recent studies indicate that people with schizophrenia are either extraordinarily sensitive to the neurotransmitter dopamine or produce too much dopamine. This theory is supported by the fact that all of the drugs used to control the psychotic symptoms of schizophrenia work by blocking certain dopamine receptors in the brain.

Schizophrenia affects men with a slightly greater frequency than women and with a somewhat worse course and prognosis. The first psychotic symptoms often appear in the teens or early twenties in men and in the late twenties or early thirties in women.

Symptoms

The classic symptoms of schizophrenia include:

- *Delusions.* Delusions are false ideas that the schizophrenic person fervently believes to be true despite all evidence to the contrary. Delusions of persecution, such as being followed and spied on by foreign terrorists, are the most common. Referential delusions—when someone believes that specific chapters of books, newspaper articles, television shows, or song lyrics are directed at him—are also common. Sometimes schizophrenic delusions take on a bizarre tone. An individual might, for example, believe that his internal organs were removed and replaced with someone else's organs or that other people can read his mind.
- *Hallucinations.* Schizophrenics hear, see, feel, or smell things that do not exist in reality. Auditory hallucinations—hearing voices—are by far the most common. Typically, the voices comment on the individual's thoughts or behavior, insult him, threaten him, or tell him what to do.
- *Disorganized speech.* The person's thought processes are chaotic and illogical, resulting in abrupt shifting from one topic to another, substituting sounds or rhymes for words, making up nonsensical words, or stringing words together randomly and incomprehensibly in a kind of "word salad."
- *Grossly disorganized or catatonic behavior.* Disorganized behavior encompasses a wide range of actions—from childlike silliness and unpredictable agitation to appearing noticeably disheveled and dressing in an unusual manner (such as wear-

ing a hat, scarf, and gloves on a hot summer day). A schizophrenic displaying catatonic behavior may be unable to move or speak, maintain a rigid pose for a long period of time, aimlessly flail his arms and legs about, senselessly mimic the movements of another person, or senselessly repeat words or phrases spoken by another person.

- *Absence of normal moods and emotions.* Victims of schizophrenia are often immobile, unresponsive, and emotionless, avoid eye contact, and display limited body language. Their "conversations" are often brief and empty. They may sit still for a long time and show little interest in working or participating in social activities. They also may exhibit inappropriate emotions, such as laughing when talking about a tragic event or displaying no emotion at all when talking about an exciting event.

These symptoms do not mean that schizophrenic individuals are completely out of touch with reality. They know, for example, that knives and forks are used for eating, clocks are used for telling time, and streets are used for driving vehicles. Schizophrenia does, however, compromise their ability to determine whether the events or situations they perceive are real. A schizophrenic person in an active phase standing in line at a supermarket, for example, may not know how to react when he hears a voice say, "You look like a mess." Is the voice coming from the person standing behind him, or is it only in his head? Is it real or a hallucination when he sees someone lying face down on the sidewalk?

The initial symptoms of schizophrenia are much more subtle—tenseness, inability to concentrate, difficulty falling asleep, and social withdrawal. As a result, family and friends may not notice them or may attribute them to "going through a phase." Eventually, however, the individual's personality, appearance, social relationships, and school or work performance begin to deteriorate. Finally, psychotic symptoms break through. Psychiatrists diagnose schizophrenia when the condition has lasted at least six months and has included an active psychotic phase.

Schizophrenia is a disease with many faces, however. Someone who suffers primarily from persecutory delusions or auditory hallucinations is said to have *paranoid schizophrenia;* a person who mainly experiences disorganized speech and behavior is said to have *disorganized schizophrenia;* an individual who exhibits motor disturbances is said to have *catatonic schizophrenia.* Because the intensity, severity, and frequency of both psychotic and remission symptoms can vary greatly from person to person, many psychiatrists use the term *schizophrenia* to describe a spectrum of illnesses that range from relatively mild to severe. Others think of schizophrenia as a collection of related disorders.

It's important to note that sometimes people develop psychotic symptoms as a result of other psychiatric illnesses or undetected medical disorders. Severe depression, manic depression, Alzheimer's disease, endocrine disorders, and seizure disorders, for example, can trigger psychotic symptoms. For this reason, a complete medical history should be taken and a complete physical examination should be performed to rule out other causes of the symptoms before concluding that a person has schizophrenia.

Treatment

The outlook for people with schizophrenia has improved dramatically over the past twenty-five years. Although a completely effective treatment still has not been discovered, antipsychotic drugs help many individuals suffering from schizophrenia improve enough to function competently and lead independent, satisfying lives.

Since chlorpromazine (Thorazine) was introduced in the early 1950s, it has been joined by more than thirty other antipsychotic drugs. Despite the fact that they differ in chemical structure, take effect at different rates, and have varying degrees of potency, they all achieve the same result—a significant reduction of delusions, hallucinations, and disorganized speech and behavior. Antipsychotic drugs also help to reduce the frequency of future psychotic episodes. With continued drug therapy, only about 40 percent of recovered individuals suffer relapses within two years of discharge from a hospital. This figure, although high, compares favorably to the 80 percent relapse rate when medication is discontinued.

In addition to chlorpromazine, commonly prescribed antipsychotic drugs include fluphenazine (Prolixin, Permitil), haloperidol (Haldol), loxapine (Loxitane), mesoridazine (Serentil), molindone (Moban), perphenazine (Trilafon), pimozide (Orap), thiothixene (Navane), thioridazine (Mellaril), and trifluoperazine (Stelazine).

Like virtually all medications, antipsychotic drugs have side effects and must be carefully monitored by a psychiatrist. During the early stages of drug therapy, individuals might be troubled by drowsiness, dizziness, faintness, dry mouth, nasal congestion, nausea, urinary retention, constipation, menstrual changes, sexual dysfunction, and blurred vision. Fortunately, most of these unwanted side effects can be corrected by lowering the dosage or controlled by other medications.

All of the antipsychotic drugs mentioned above can also produce major movement side effects. Within hours or days of beginning drug therapy, some people experience sudden, severe, and painful spasms of the muscles in the head and neck. This frightening condition, called *acute dystonia,* can be reversed almost immediately with an injection of the proper antidote. To prevent it from occurring, many psychiatrists prescribe antipsychotic drugs and antidotes simultaneously.

Parkinsonian syndrome mimics the symptoms of Parkinson's disease—a tremor or shaking of the hands, masklike facial expression, slowed body movements, rigidity of the joints, drooling, and shuffling walk. These side effects typically set in days to weeks after the start of antipsychotic drug therapy and respond well to the same medications that are used to treat acute dystonia.

As many as 75 percent of people who take antipsychotic drugs also develop some degree of agitated restlessness called *akathisia.* Individuals experiencing akathisia constantly feel like moving and are unable to sit still. This sensation of internal restlessness is often uncomfortable and aggravating enough to make people want to "jump out of their skin." Unfortunately, it can be difficult to treat. Switching to another antipsychotic drug or taking the beta-blocker propranolol (Inderal), which is used to treat high blood pressure, may provide some relief. Not surprisingly, akathisia is the number one reason that schizophrenic individuals stop taking antipsychotic drugs.

A much more serious, and often unavoidable, side effect of antipsychotic drugs is *tardive dyskinesia* (TD). This neurological syndrome, which is characterized by involuntary movements of the mouth, lips, and tongue, affects at least 20 percent and possibly up to 50 percent of people taking antipsychotic medications. It often begins with small tongue tremors, facial tics, and abnormal jaw movements, which may progress into protruding and rolling of the tongue, lip licking and smacking, chewing or sucking motions, puckering of the cheeks, pouting, and grimacing. Sometimes, spasmodic movements of the hands, feet, arms, legs, neck, and shoulders also take place.

Most people do not begin to show symptoms of TD until they have been taking antipsychotic drugs for many years. Symptoms can emerge earlier, however, especially in the elderly since being forty-five or more years old is one of the major risk factors. Women and individuals on high-dose therapy also seem to be at increased risk of developing the disorder.

Because there is no cure for tardive dyskinesia and its effects can be permanent, psychiatrists focus on prevention. People taking antipsychotic drugs should be carefully examined every six months for early signs of the syndrome. As an added precaution, psychiatrists should prescribe antipsychotic medications at the lowest possible effective doses or for the shortest possible time. If symptoms appear despite these preventive measures, drug therapy may have to be discontinued unless the medication is absolutely vital to the individual. Switching to clozapine, a different type of antipsychotic drug, is another alternative (see page 188). To reduce the risk in people with chronic schizophrenia, many psychopharmacologists recommend reducing dosage levels.

Neuroleptic malignant syndrome (NMS) is a rare

but potentially life-threatening side effect characterized by severe muscle rigidity throughout the body. Other features of NMS include high fever, rapid heartbeat, rapid breathing, excessive perspiration, abnormal blood pressure, and kidney failure. Neuroleptic malignant syndrome is a major medical emergency requiring immediate hospitalization, discontinuation of all antipsychotic medications, administration of antidotes, and cooling of the entire body in the event of a high fever.

Differences among antipsychotic drugs. As mentioned earlier, all antipsychotic drugs help to control the psychotic symptoms of schizophrenia. The main difference between one medication and another is the side effects that it typically produces. Low-potency antipsychotics—chlorpromazine, loxapine, molindone, and thioridazine—tend to lower blood pressure and cause sedation as their main side effects. High-potency antipsychotics—fluphenazine, haloperidol, perphenazine, pimozide, thiothixene, and trifluoperazine—tend to produce more major movement side effects such as acute dystonia, parkinsonian symptoms, and akathisia.

For people who do not respond to traditional antipsychotic drugs or cannot tolerate the side effects, clozapine (Clozaril) is often an effective alternative. Scientific studies have shown that clozapine produces significant improvements in 30 to 60 percent of "treatment-resistant" or "neuroleptic refractory" schizophrenics. It also does not appear to cause acute dystonia, parkinsonian syndrome, akathisia, or tardive dyskinesia.

Although the antipsychotic properties of clozapine were first discovered more than twenty-five years ago, it did not become widely available in the United

States until 1990. One of the main reasons for the delay is a potentially fatal side effect of the drug called *agranulocytosis,* which results in the failure of the body to produce certain white blood cells. Fortunately, the condition is reversible if detected in its early stages. Since agranulocytosis can strike without warning, however, clozapine is prescribed only to individuals who comply with mandatory weekly blood tests. Other potential side effects include rapid heartbeat, low blood pressure, sedation, fever, nausea and vomiting, constipation, dry mouth, and increased salivation. Clozapine also carries a slight risk of seizures. If necessary, it can be administered along with an antiseizure medication.

Risperidone (Risperdal), which was recently approved by the Food and Drug Administration for the treatment of schizophrenia, also does not seem to produce acute dystonia, parkinsonian syndrome, or akathisia if administered at an optimal therapeutic dose. The most common side effects include anxiety, drowsiness, dizziness, constipation, nausea, indigestion, rhinitis, rash, and rapid heartbeat. Risperidone has also been shown to control negative symptoms of the illness—apathy, social withdrawal, lack of motivation, and blunted emotional response—much more effectively than traditional antipsychotic drugs. Consequently, it may become the drug of choice for the treatment of schizophrenia in the near future. But it is too early to tell whether risperidone, like clozapine, will be effective in treating neuroleptic refractory schizophrenia or whether it will cause tardive dyskinesia. Both clozapine and risperidone block the neurotransmitter serotonin in addition to dopamine. Other combined serotonin-dopamine antagonists (SDAs) are currently being developed.

Since antipsychotic drugs are associated with so many side effects and risks, it is not unusual for "outsiders" to wonder why schizophrenic individuals bother to take medication. To the millions of victims and family members who live with this debilitating disease, the answer is obvious. The benefits of antipsychotic drugs—relief from crippling breakdowns and the opportunity to once again be an active participant at school, at work, at home, and in the community—far outweigh the risks.

Questions & Answers

Q. Is there a cure for schizophrenia?

A. Unfortunately, there is no cure for schizophrenia at present. Antipsychotic drugs *control* the condition the way insulin controls diabetes, but they don't *cure* it. Like diabetics, schizophrenics often need to be under medical care for the rest of their lives. Ten to 30 percent, however, recover late in life.

Q. How common is suicide among people with schizophrenia?

A. People with schizophrenia have a higher rate of suicide than the general population. Approximately 10 percent of schizophrenic individuals commit suicide, particularly men under the age of thirty who are unemployed, display symptoms of depression, and have been discharged from the hospital recently.

Q. Are people with schizophrenia violent?

A. Although the news media tends to link criminal violence with mental illness, most people with schizophrenia are not violent. More typically, they prefer to withdraw and be left alone. It's generally agreed that most violent crimes are not committed by schizophrenic individuals and that most schizophrenic individuals do not commit violent crimes.

Q. Will I have to take medication for the rest of my life?
A. That's a difficult question to answer. If you have chronic schizophrenia, you probably *will* need to take antipsychotic drugs for the rest of your life. If you stop taking your medication, the psychotic episodes will undoubtedly return. On the other hand, if the psychotic episodes occur years apart or if you experience only one episode, you may not need to be on medication continuously. Since the course of schizophrenia is hard to predict, however, it's important to discuss all the options with your psychiatrist before deciding to stop taking your medication.

Q. What can be done for people who forget or refuse to take their medication?
A. It can be difficult to convince certain schizophrenic people that they need to take medication, particularly when they begin to feel better. One solution is to prescribe injections of long-acting antipsychotic drugs. Prolixin Decanoate can be injected once every two weeks; Haldol Decanoate can be injected once every two to four weeks.

Q. Will antipsychotic drugs alone help me get my life back in order?
A. Medication helps to relieve psychotic symptoms such as hallucinations, delusions, and incoherence. Some of the newer drugs such as clozapine and

risperidone also may treat negative symptoms such as blunted emotional response and decreased interest. No medication, however, will solve the personal problems that most likely have cropped up as a result of the psychotic episodes. If schizophrenia has taken its toll on your family life, schoolwork, career path, self-esteem, or ability to establish and maintain relationships with others, for example, you'll most likely benefit from psychosocial therapy. Options include individual psychotherapy, family therapy, social and vocational training, and self-help groups. Keep in mind, however, that it's impossible to "talk yourself out of" schizophrenia. Psychotherapy should always be viewed as a supplement to, not a replacement for, medication.

Sleep Disorders

For most of us, falling asleep is easy. After a long, hard day on the job, at school, or at home with the kids, we're down for the count within minutes of slipping under the covers. Getting out of bed when the alarm clock rings is our only sleep-related "problem." For more than one-third of Americans, however, falling asleep is a nightmare.

People who suffer from insomnia—the inability to get enough sleep—approach bedtime with apprehension. They imagine the hours and hours of lying awake, tossing and turning, wondering when sleep will come, worrying about the problem, and anticipating how sluggish, exhausted, and irritable they'll feel in the morning.

Insomnia, by far the most common sleep disorder, takes on many forms. The most common are difficulty falling asleep (taking more than thirty to forty-five minutes), waking up frequently during the night, and waking up early and not being able to get back to sleep. Young adults usually have trouble falling asleep; middle-aged and elderly adults are more likely to have difficulty with staying asleep and waking up early. Insomnia can begin at any age and last for a few days (transient insomnia), a few weeks (short-term insomnia), or indefinitely (long-term insomnia).

Transient insomnia, which affects nearly everyone from time to time, is often triggered by a specific mental or physical stress—the first day at a new school or job, a final exam, an important business meeting, an argument with a spouse, a bad cold, headache, toothache, backache, sore muscles, indigestion, or airline travel involving time-zone changes.

Short-term insomnia often crops up during periods of ongoing stress—moving to a new house or city, financial difficulties, marital problems, divorce, the death of a loved one, losing a job, looking for a new job, or retirement.

Long-term insomnia is sometimes caused by environmental factors such as living near an airport or on a noisy street or working a night shift. More often, however, it is a symptom of a more serious medical or psychiatric condition such as depression, generalized anxiety disorder, manic depression, premenstrual syndrome, post-traumatic stress disorder, schizophrenia, congestive heart failure, diabetes, emphysema, epilepsy, hepatitis, multiple sclerosis, or tuberculosis.

For this reason, anyone suffering from insomnia should undergo a complete physical examination before beginning treatment.

In this chapter, we'll also discuss narcolepsy, sleep apnea, and nocturnal myoclonus.

Treatment

Most health professionals agree that treatment for insomnia should begin with "sleep hygiene therapy" rather than prescription or over-the-counter sleep medications. The following simple measures have cured even the most chronic cases of insomnia. Give them a try before visiting your family physician or local pharmacy.

- Stop taking daytime naps.
- Stop smoking. Nicotine raises blood pressure and pulse rate, both of which can make it difficult to fall asleep.
- Stop consuming caffeine after midday. In addition to coffee, the most obvious culprit, caffeine is found in tea, cocoa, chocolate, and many cola drinks.
- Do exercise during the late afternoon or early evening to improve your chances of falling asleep. Since exercise is temporarily stimulating, however, avoid working out within three hours of bedtime.
- Avoid alcohol. A beer or glass of wine before bedtime will most likely make you sleepy, but it will also most likely wake you up with a sudden jolt several hours later when the relaxing effect wears off.

- Don't eat a heavy meal before bedtime. Digestion can keep you awake.
- Avoid drinking liquids close to bedtime so that you won't wake up during the night to urinate.
- Make sure your sleep environment is comfortable. Your pillow and mattress, as well as the temperature of your bedroom, should be conducive to getting a good night's rest. If barking dogs, car alarms, or your partner's snoring are a problem, invest in a pair of earplugs or a "white noise" generator. If the morning light bothers you, wear a sleeping mask.
- Try to go to bed at the same time every night—even on weekends. Staying up late on Saturday night and sleeping in on Sunday can set your body clock forward a few hours, creating what researchers call "Sunday-night insomnia."
- Release the stress of the day when you get into bed by alternately tensing and relaxing each muscle in your body, breathing deeply, or visualizing a peaceful scene.
- If you can't fall asleep within fifteen minutes, get up and do something else until you feel tired. Follow the same advice if you wake up during the night and can't fall back to sleep.

Drug therapy. If these measures don't work, drug therapy is often the next step. Benzodiazepines are the most frequently prescribed sleep medications. They speed the onset of sleep, reduce the number of nighttime awakenings, and increase total sleep time. The five benzodiazepines used specifically for insomnia are estazolam (ProSom), flurazepam (Dalmane), quazepam (Doral), temazepam (Restoril), and triazolam (Halcion).

Flurazepam is a long-acting benzodiazepine, meaning it remains in the body for at least a day. Consequently, it may cause "hangover" side effects such as drowsiness, dizziness, and light-headedness. Quazepam, a relatively new long-acting benzodiazepine, doesn't appear to cause such adverse effects. Estazolam and temazepam, which remain active for about ten hours, are also less likely to cause daytime drowsiness. Triazolam, an extremely short-acting benzodiazepine, is eliminated from the body in about six hours. As a result, it rarely produces morning-after drowsiness. It does, however, cause morning-after memory loss in some people.

The Food and Drug Administration recently approved a new type of short-acting sleep medication called zolpidem (Ambien). According to the manufacturer, this nonbenzodiazepine sleeping pill causes little or no daytime drowsiness. However, there's not yet enough scientific evidence to support this claim. Zolpidem may very well have major advantages over the benzodiazepines, but it will take several more years of research and clinical experience to know for sure.

One potential drawback to the benzodiazepines is that they can lead to dependency, meaning the body becomes used to them and can't fall asleep without them. Some people who take benzodiazepines continuously for two weeks or more experience "rebound insomnia" when they stop using the drugs. Rebound insomnia is a bad case of insomnia that lingers until a normal sleep pattern is reestablished—usually a few nights. The longer benzodiazepines are used, the more pronounced the rebound insomnia will be. Consequently, sleeping pills should be taken sparingly, for the shortest possible stretch of time, and in the lowest effective dose. Users should also try to fall asleep on their own for at least an hour before taking a sleeping pill.

Barbiturates, highly potent drugs including phenobarbital and secobarbital, are still sometimes used in the short-term treatment of insomnia for people who can't tolerate benzodiazepines. It's important to note, however, that barbiturates are addictive, produce a high rate of mental confusion, often impair coordination, can trigger anger and depression, and can be lethal when combined with alcohol or taken in overdose. For these reasons, psychiatrists are reluctant to prescribe them.

A word about over-the-counter sleep medications: Taking them for a night or two at the recommended dosage is probably harmless. (Most contain antihistamines, which cause drowsiness in addition to relieving allergies and rashes.) However, studies show that they quickly lose their effectiveness. Furthermore, many psychiatrists maintain that over-the-counter sleeping pills cause more side effects than benzodiazepine sleeping pills and are just as likely to become habit-forming if taken for several consecutive weeks. The bottom line? If you need medication for insomnia, a prescription is preferable.

Narcolepsy

At the opposite end of the sleep-disorder spectrum is narcolepsy, a neurological condition that causes an estimated 250,000 Americans to fall asleep involuntarily. Although it is a relatively rare illness, its effects can be devastating and debilitating. Narcolepsy can, for example, seriously interfere with a person's ability to drive, hold down a job, stay in school, perform everyday tasks, engage in social activities, and maintain personal relationships.

Although this illness has been studied extensively, the exact cause remains unknown. It seems, however, to stem from a defect in the part of the central nervous system that controls sleep and wakefulness. Narcolepsy can strike at any age, but it usually begins in the early teens. Symptoms can appear all at once or develop gradually over many years.

The most common symptoms of narcolepsy are:

- *Excessive daytime sleepiness.* In most cases, EDS is the only symptom of narcolepsy. In other cases, it's the first symptom. People with the disorder often feel tired all the time. They tend to fall asleep not only in situations in which many normal people would fall asleep (after a heavy meal or during a boring lecture), but also in situations in which most people would remain awake (while eating a meal or carrying on a conversation). Sudden attacks of sleep can also strike at dangerous times (while crossing a street, driving a car, or operating machinery).
- *Cataplexy,* brief attacks of loss of muscle control, usually develops several years after EDS. Attacks can range from a momentary feeling of weakness in the knees to complete physical collapse. Cataplexy is usually triggered by stress or an intense emotion such as laughter, anger, or surprise. Sometimes attacks can be triggered by simply remembering or anticipating an emotional situation.
- *Sleep paralysis* also produces a temporary loss of muscle control. Typically, a person finds himself unable to move or speak when he is either waking up or falling asleep. Touching the individual usually makes the paralysis disappear.

- *Hypnagogic hallucinations* are vivid, dreamlike experiences that are difficult to distinguish from reality. They can be especially frightening because they occur when the person is awake.

Although narcolepsy can't be cured, it can be effectively controlled through a combination of drug therapy and behavior modification. Psychiatrists and neurologists almost always prescribe stimulants such as methylphenidate (Ritalin), dextroamphetamine (Dexedrine), or pemoline (Cylert) to combat daytime sleepiness. The most common side effects of these medications include headache, irritability, nervousness, weight loss, insomnia, gastrointestinal complaints, and palpitations.

The behavior-modification portion of the treatment plan involves making lifestyle adjustments:

- going to bed and waking up at the same time every day
- taking short naps during the day whenever necessary
- increasing physical activity
- avoiding boring or repetitive tasks
- scheduling activities that can be dangerous (such as driving, swimming, or cooking) for times when you know you'll be alert

Other Sleep Disorders

Two other sleep disorders, *sleep apnea* and *nocturnal myoclonus,* also can cause daytime sleepiness. People suffering from sleep apnea actually stop breathing dozens, sometimes hundreds, of times a night due to airway obstruction. As a result, they wake up dozens or hundreds of times a night. But, since these episodes only last a few seconds, most individuals don't even realize that their sleep has been interrupted. They do, however, feel tired and unrefreshed the following day. In addition to daytime sleepiness, symptoms of sleep apnea include loud snores or gasps alternating with periods of silence, moaning or mumbling, whole-body movements, and early-morning headaches.

Most cases are mild and don't require treatment. Severe cases may benefit from a procedure called continuous positive airway pressure, which keeps the breathing passages open during the night with a steady stream of air delivered through a mask worn over the nose and mouth. Surgery is another option for severe cases of the disorder. One procedure widens the throat. Another, used rarely, is to make a small hole at the base of the neck, below and in front of the Adam's apple. At night, a valve on a tube inserted into the hole is opened so that air can flow directly to the lungs, bypassing the blockage. During the day, the valve is closed, allowing the individual to breathe and speak normally.

People suffering from nocturnal myoclonus experience involuntary leg muscle jerks or twitches during the night. Like sleep apnea, these brief movements may cause hundreds of brief awakenings during the night and result in fatigue the following day. Some people also complain of an itching sensation in their legs, like a "current going through them," when they wake up in the morning. Treatment may involve sleeping pills, pain-relieving medications, vitamin and mineral supplements, evening exercise and/or warm baths.

Questions & Answers

Q. Does everyone need eight hours of sleep?

A. Most adults *do* sleep between seven and eight hours, but there are many exceptions to the rule. A "short sleeper" may need only three or four hours and actually function worse with more sleep. A "long sleeper," on the other hand, may need more than ten hours. "Variable sleepers" seem to need more sleep at times of stress and less during peaceful times. You know you're getting the right amount of sleep if you're able to stay awake and alert during the day.

Q. Does the amount of sleep a person needs change with age?

A. Definitely. A newborn infant may sleep sixteen hours a day, an adolescent may sleep very deeply for nine or ten consecutive hours, and an elderly person may only sleep five or six hours a night. It's common, and perfectly normal, to sleep less as you get older.

Q. Are benzodiazepines addicting?

A. The term *addiction* really doesn't apply to benzodiazepines. People who are addicted to a drug are completely consumed by it and will do anything to get their hands on it. People who take benzodiazepine sleeping pills definitely do *not* display that type of behavior. It's more accurate to say that benzodiazepine sleeping pills can be habit-forming. People who take them for an extended period can become dependent upon them, have a great deal of trouble falling asleep without them, and as a result, find it difficult to stop taking them.

Q. Can I die from an overdose of benzodiazepines?

A. While it's true that benzodiazepines are often used in suicide attempts, attempts made with benzodiazepines alone are rarely fatal. Unless you combine benzodiazepines with alcohol or other drugs, particularly barbiturates, you're not likely to die from an overdose. You're more likely to become very drowsy or stuporous or fall into a deep sleep. If you experience any of these symptoms, you should be taken to the nearest hospital emergency room immediately.

Q. What are the consequences of insomnia?

A. Chronic insomnia can have devastating effects on the careers and lives of those afflicted with it. Insomniacs, for example, have twice as many car accidents as noninsomniacs. They also spend about half as much time working and studying as noninsomniacs. Some insomniacs suffer from impaired memory and cognitive functioning, and poor interpersonal and coping skills. Others are simply dismissed as lazy.

Q. Is narcolepsy hereditary?

A. Studies show that first-degree relatives (parents and siblings) of a person with narcolepsy are about eight times more likely to develop some disorder of excessive sleepiness than the general population. Members of families with a history of narcolepsy often start to display symptoms at around the same age.

Q. How would you know you have sleep apnea if you don't even know you're waking up during the night?

A. The telltale signs of sleep apnea—loud snoring, gasping, moaning, or mumbling, and whole-body movements—are usually pointed out by a bed partner or roommate.

Q. Is it possible to have sleep apnea and still breathe normally while you're awake?
A. Definitely. Excessive relaxation of the muscles used for breathing or trouble with the brain's control over breathing may only take place during sleep.

Q. Are sleep disorders more common in older people?
A. Sleep apnea *does* become more common with age. The periodic leg movements associated with nocturnal myoclonus also tend to become more frequent and severe as people grow older.

4

Psychiatric Drug Profiles

Alprazolam

Brand Name
Xanax

General Information
Alprazolam is used in the treatment of anxiety disorder, panic disorder, and anxiety associated with depression. It is a member of the class of drugs called benzodiazepines, which facilitate the action of the neurotransmitter GABA (gamma-aminobutyric acid). At lower doses, alprazolam decreases anxiety. At higher doses, it causes sedation and sleep. Alprazolam relaxes skeletal muscles as well.

Symptoms of anxiety include trembling, twitching, heart palpitations, shortness of breath, sweaty palms, clammy skin, dry mouth, dizziness, nausea, and trouble swallowing.

Side Effects

Side effects usually appear at the beginning of treatment and disappear with continued use of the medication.

More common side effects may include abdominal discomfort; abnormal involuntary movement; agitation; allergies; anxiety; blurred vision; chest pain; confusion; constipation; decreased or increased sex drive; depression; diarrhea; difficulty urinating; dizziness; dream abnormalities; drowsiness; dry mouth; fainting; fatigue; fear; fluid retention; headache; hyperventilation; impaired memory; increased or decreased appetite; increased or decreased salivation; infection; insomnia; irritability; light-headedness; low blood pressure; menstrual problems; muscle cramps; muscular twitching; nausea and vomiting; nervousness; palpitations; perspiration; rapid heartbeat; rash; restlessness; ringing in the ears; sexual dysfunction; skin inflammation; sleepiness; speech difficulties; stiffness; stuffy nose; talkativeness; tingling sensation; tremors; uninhibited behavior; upper respiratory infections; warm feeling; weakness; and weight gain or loss.

Less common or rare side effects may include abnormal muscle tone; decreased coordination; difficulty concentrating; double vision; hallucinations; itching; loss of appetite; rage; sedation; seizures; sleep disturbances; slurred speech; spastic muscles; stimulation; taste disturbances; temporary memory loss; urinary retention; weakness in the muscles and bones; and yellowing of the skin and whites of the eyes.

If you experience any of these side effects or reactions, notify your doctor as soon as possible.

Important Precautions

Do not take alprazolam if you have narrow-angle glaucoma or if you have ever had an allergic reaction or hypersensitivity to alprazolam or a similar drug.

Alprazolam may make you drowsy or less alert. Do not drive, operate machinery, or participate in any high-risk activities until you know exactly how the drug affects you.

Abruptly discontinuing alprazolam may result in withdrawal symptoms such as blurred vision, decreased concentration, decreased mental clarity, diarrhea, heightened awareness of noise or bright lights, impaired sense of smell, loss of appetite, muscle cramps, seizures, tingling sensation, twitching, and weight loss. When ending treatment with this medication, follow your doctor's schedule for a gradual withdrawal.

Food and Drug Interactions

If alprazolam is taken with certain other drugs, the effects of either drug could be increased, decreased, or changed. Before beginning treatment with alprazolam, tell your doctor if you are taking any other prescription or over-the-counter medications.

It is particularly important to check with your doctor before combining alprazolam with other central nervous system depressants, other psychotropic drugs, oral contraceptives, cimetidine (Tagamet), desipramine (Norpramin), or imipramine (Tofranil).

Do not drink alcohol while taking alprazolam.

Recommended Dosage

The recommended daily dosage of alprazolam depends upon whether it is being used to treat anxiety disorder or panic disorder.

Anxiety Disorder

Usual dosage for adults: The usual starting dose is .25 to .5 mg three times a day. If necessary, this amount may be gradually increased to a maximum of 4 mg a day taken in several divided doses.

Panic Disorder

Usual dosage for adults: The usual starting dosage is .5 mg three times a day. If necessary, this amount may be gradually increased by increments of 1 mg until an effective dose is reached. The average dose is 5 to 6 mg a day.

Dosages for the elderly should be determined by a doctor.

The safety and effectiveness of alprazolam in children under the age of eighteen has not been established.

Overdosage

An overdose of alprazolam, either alone or combined with alcohol, can be fatal. Symptoms of overdose may include coma, confusion, impaired coordination, sleepiness, and slowed reflexes. If you experience any of these symptoms, go to the nearest hospital emergency room immediately.

Pregnancy and Lactation

Alprazolam is associated with an increased risk of respiratory problems and muscular weakness in newborn babies. As a result, it should not be taken during pregnancy. If you are pregnant or plan to become pregnant, notify your doctor immediately.

The drug may pass into breast milk and may be harmful to a nursing infant. If the medication is essential to your health, your doctor may advise you not to breast-feed while you are taking it.

Amitriptyline

Brand Names

Elavil, Endep

General Information

Amitriptyline is used in the treatment of depression. It is a member of the class of drugs called tricyclic antidepressants, which work by blocking the reabsorption of the neurotransmitters serotonin, norepinephrine, and dopamine in the brain. This suggests that many of the symptoms of depression may result from imbalances of one or more of these neurotransmitters.

Symptoms of depression include low, anxious, or "empty" feelings; loss of interest and pleasure in activities previously enjoyed; noticeable change of appetite; noticeable change in sleeping patterns; fatigue or loss of energy; feelings of hopelessness or pessimism; feelings of guilt, worthlessness, or helplessness; inability to concentrate, make decisions, or remember details; recurring thoughts of death or suicide, wishing to die or attempting suicide; and aches and pains, constipation, or other physical ailments that cannot be explained.

Side Effects

Side effects may include abnormal movements; anxiety; black tongue; blurred vision; breast development in males; breast enlargement; coma; confusion; constipation; delusions; diarrhea; dilated pupils; disorientation; disturbed concentration; dizziness or light-headedness; drowsiness; dry mouth; excessive or spontaneous flow of milk; excitement; fatigue; fluid retention; frequent or difficult urination; hair loss; hallucinations; headache; heart attack; hepatitis; high fever; high or low blood sugar; hives; impotence; increased or decreased sex drive; increased perspiration; increased pressure in the eyes; inflammation of the mouth; intestinal blockage; irregular heartbeat; lack or loss of coordination; loss of appetite; nausea; numbness; rapid or pounding heartbeat; rash; reddish or purplish spots on the skin; restlessness; ringing in the ears; sensitivity to light; speech difficulty; stomach upset; strange taste in mouth; stroke; swelling in the face and tongue; swelling of the testicles; tingling; tremors; urinary retention; vomiting; weakness; and weight gain or loss.

If you experience any of these side effects or reactions, notify your doctor as soon as possible.

Important Precautions

In general, you should not take amitriptyline if you are recovering from a heart attack, if you are taking another type of antidepressant called a monoamine oxidase inhibitor (MAOI) or have taken one within the past two weeks, or if you have ever had an allergic reaction or hypersensitivity to amitriptyline or a similar drug.

Use this medication with caution if you have a history of cardiovascular or thyroid disease, glaucoma, or other chronic eye conditions, seizures, or urinary retention.

Amitriptyline may make you feel dizzy and drowsy. Do not drive, operate machinery, or participate in any high-risk activities until you know exactly how the drug affects you. It might also make you feel dizzy or light-headed when getting up from a seated or prone position. If getting up slowly doesn't solve this problem, notify your doctor.

Abruptly discontinuing amitriptyline may result in headaches, nausea, and other unpleasant side effects. When ending treatment with this drug, follow your doctor's schedule for a gradual withdrawal.

Food and Drug Interactions

If amitriptyline is taken with certain other drugs, the effects of either drug could be increased, decreased, or changed. Before beginning treatment with amitriptyline, tell your doctor if you are taking any other prescription or over-the-counter medications.

Amitriptyline should not be combined with MAOIs. It is also important to check with your doctor before combining amitriptyline with allergy and cold medications, anticholinergic drugs such as Artane and Cogentin, antihistamines, antipsychotic drugs, barbiturates, estrogen, muscle relaxants, oral contraceptives, sedative or hypnotic drugs, seizure medications, thyroid medications, albuterol (Proventil, Ventolin), cimetidine (Tagamet), disulfiram (Antabuse), ethchlorvynol (Placidyl), fluoxetine (Prozac), or guanethidine (Ismelin).

Amitriptyline should not be taken with alcohol, sleeping pills, tranquilizers, or narcotic painkillers.

Recommended Dosage

Usual dosage for adults: 50 to 150 mg a day taken in several divided doses with a total daily limit of 300 mg.

Usual dosage for adolescents and the elderly: 10 mg taken three times a day plus an additional 20 mg taken at bedtime.

Amitriptyline is not recommended for children under the age of twelve.

Overdosage

An overdose of amitriptyline can be fatal. Symptoms of overdose may include abnormally low blood pressure, congestive heart failure, convulsions, dilated pupils, drowsiness, rapid or irregular heartbeat, reduced body temperature, and unresponsiveness or coma. Other warning signs include agitation, excessive movement, extremely high body temperature, flush over the entire body, rigid muscles, and vomiting. If you experience any of these symptoms, go to the nearest hospital emergency room immediately.

153

Pregnancy and Lactation

The safety of amitriptyline use during pregnancy has not been established. If you are pregnant or plan to become pregnant, notify your doctor immediately.

The drug passes into breast milk and may be harmful to a nursing infant. If the medication is essential to your health, your doctor may advise you not to breast-feed while you are taking it.

Amoxapine

Brand Name

Asendin

General Information

Amoxapine is used in the treatment of depression with or without anxiety or agitation. It has a mild sedative effect. Amoxapine works by blocking the presynaptic reuptake of the neurotransmitters serotonin, norepinephrine, and dopamine in the brain. This suggests that many of the symptoms of depression may result from imbalances of one or more of these neurotransmitters.

Symptoms of depression include low, anxious, or "empty" feelings; loss of interest and pleasure in activities previously enjoyed; noticeable change of appetite; noticeable change in sleeping patterns; fatigue or loss of energy; feelings of hopelessness or pessimism; feelings of guilt, worthlessness, or helplessness; inability to concentrate, make decisions, or remember details; recurring thoughts of death or suicide, wishing to die or attempting suicide; and aches and pains, constipation, or other physical ailments that cannot be explained.

Side Effects

Amoxapine has the potential to cause a serious and at times permanent side effect called tardive dyskinesia. This neurological syndrome results in involuntary movements of the mouth, lips, and tongue such as tongue rolling, lip licking and smacking, chewing or sucking motions, pouting, and grimacing.

Some people have developed neuroleptic malignant syndrome while taking amoxapine. This potentially life-threatening condition is characterized by altered mental state, extremely high body temperature, rigid muscles, and irregular blood pressure, heartbeat, and pulse. For these reasons, amoxapine is not usually prescribed.

More common side effects may include anxiety; blurred vision; confusion; dizziness; drowsiness; dry mouth; excitement; fatigue; fluid retention; headache, increased appetite; increased perspiration; insomnia; lack of muscle coordination; nausea; nervousness; nightmares; pounding heartbeat; restlessness; skin rash; tremors; and weakness.

Less common or rare side effects may include abdominal pain; blood disorders; breast enlargement; diarrhea; difficulty urinating; dilated pupils; disorientation; disturbed concentration; excessive or spontaneous flow of milk; extremely high body temperature; fainting; fever; gas; high or low blood pressure; hives;

impotence; increased or decreased sex drive; itching; lack of coordination; menstrual irregularity; numbness; painful ejaculation; rapid heartbeat; ringing in the ears; seizures; sensitivity to light; strange taste in mouth; stuffy nose; tingling sensation in arms and legs; upset stomach; vomiting; watery eyes; and weight gain or loss.

If you experience any of these side effects or reactions, notify your doctor as soon as possible.

Important Precautions

Keep in mind that amoxapine can cause tardive dyskinesia and neuroleptic malignant syndrome.

In general, you should not take amoxapine if you are recovering from a heart attack, if you are taking another type of antidepressant called a monoamine oxidase inhibitor (MAOI), or if you have ever had an allergic reaction or hypersensitivity to amoxapine or a similar drug.

Use this medication with caution if you have a history of heart disease, seizures, urinary retention, narrow-angle glaucoma, or increased eye pressure.

Amoxapine may make you feel dizzy and drowsy. Do not drive, operate machinery, or participate in any high-risk activities until you know exactly how the drug affects you.

Food and Drug Interactions

If amoxapine is taken with certain other drugs, the effects of either drug could be increased, decreased, or changed. Before beginning treatment with amoxapine, tell your doctor if you are taking any other prescription or over-the-counter medications.

Amoxapine should not be combined with MAOIs. It is also important to check with your doctor before taking amoxapine with albuterol (Ventolin, Proventil), cimetidine (Tagamet), anticholinergic drugs, barbiturates, sedatives, or other central nervous system depressants.

Do not drink alcohol while taking amoxapine.

Recommended Dosage

Usual dosage for adults: The usual starting dose is 50 mg taken two or three times a day. This amount may be increased to 100 mg two or three times a day by the end of the first week of treatment. Dosages above 300 mg a day are not recommended unless lower dosages have failed to produce adequate results during a trial period of at least two weeks. When an effective dosage is reached, the medication may be taken in a single dose at bedtime.

Usual dosage for the elderly: The usual starting dose is 25 mg taken two or three times a day. This amount may be increased to 50 mg two or three times a day by the end of the first week of treatment.

The safety and effectiveness of amoxapine use in children under the age of sixteen has not been established.

Overdosage

Symptoms of an amoxapine overdose may include coma, convulsions, kidney failure, and prolonged seizures requiring medical attention. If you experience any of these symptoms, go to the nearest hospital emergency room immediately.

Pregnancy and Lactation

The safety of amoxapine use during pregnancy has not been established. As a result, it should only be taken during pregnancy if the potential benefits clearly outweigh any potential risks to the fetus. If you are pregnant or plan to become pregnant, notify your doctor immediately.

The drug passes into breast milk and may be harmful to a nursing infant. If the medication is essential to your health, your doctor may advise you not to breast-feed while you are taking it.

Bupropion

Brand Name
Wellbutrin

General Information

Bupropion is used to treat depression. It tends to have somewhat of a stimulant effect. While no one knows exactly how it works, it may work via effects on the neurotransmitters norepinephrine and dopamine. This suggests that many of the symptoms of depression may result from imbalances of one or both of these neurotransmitters.

Symptoms of depression include low, anxious, or "empty" feelings; loss of interest and pleasure in activities previously enjoyed; noticeable change of appetite; noticeable change in sleeping patterns; fatigue or loss of energy; feelings of hopelessness or pessimism; feelings of guilt, worthlessness, or helplessness; inability to concentrate, make decisions, or remember details; recurring thoughts of death or suicide, wishing to die or attempting suicide; and aches and pains, constipation, or other physical ailments that cannot be explained.

Side Effects

Seizures occur in approximately four out of every thousand people taking bupropion.

More common side effects may include agitation, constipation, dizziness, dry mouth, excessive perspiration, headache, nausea, skin rash, sleep disturbances, tremors, and vomiting.

Other side effects may include acne; bed-wetting; blurred vision; chest pain; chills; complete or nearly complete loss of movement; confusion; difficulty breathing; dry skin; episodes of elation, irritability, or overactivity; extreme calmness; fatigue; fever; fluid retention; flulike symptoms; gum irritation and inflammation; hair color changes; hair loss; hives; impotence; increased sex drive; indigestion; itching; lack of coordination and clumsiness; menstrual complaints; mood instability; muscle rigidity; painful ejaculation; painful erection; retarded ejaculation; ringing in the ears; sexual dysfunction; suicidal thoughts; thirst; toothache; urinary disturbances; and weight gain or loss.

If you experience any of these side effects or reactions, notify your doctor as soon as possible.

Important Precautions

Do not take bupropion if you have any type of seizure disorder, if you have a history of anorexia or bulimia, if you are taking another type of antidepressant called a monoamine oxidase inhibitor (MAOI) or have taken one within the past two weeks, or if you have ever had an allergic reaction or hypersensitivity to bupropion or a similar drug.

Do not take other medications that might cause seizures.

Approximately 28 percent of people who take bupropion lose five pounds or more. If you have already lost weight due to depression, and if further weight loss would be harmful to your health, bupropion may not be the right antidepressant for you.

Bupropion may impair your coordination. Do not drive, operate machinery, or participate in any high-risk activities until you know exactly how the drug affects you.

Food and Drug Interactions

If bupropion is taken with certain other drugs, the effects of either drug could be increased, decreased, or changed. Before beginning treatment with bupropion, tell your doctor if you are taking any other prescription or over-the-counter medications.

Combining bupropion with a MAOI can lead to a sudden, potentially life-threatening increase in blood pressure. If you have been taking a MAOI, you must wait at least two weeks after discontinuing therapy with the drug before starting therapy with bupropion.

It is also important to check with your doctor

before combining bupropion with antipsychotics, tricyclic antidepressants, phenobarbital, carbamazepine (Tegretol), cimetidine (Tagamet), levodopa (Larodopa), or phenytoin (Dilantin).

Do not drink alcohol while taking bupropion.

Recommended Dosage

Usual dosage for adults: The usual starting dose is 200 mg a day taken in two divided doses. This amount may be increased to 300 mg a day taken in three divided doses with at least six hours between doses. If no improvement is observed after several weeks of treatment at 300 mg a day, your doctor may increase the daily dose to 450 mg taken in three divided doses with at least six hours between doses.

Dosages for the elderly should be determined by a doctor.

Bupropion is not recommended for children under the age of eighteen.

Overdosage

Symptoms of a bupropion overdose may include hallucinations, heart failure, loss of consciousness, rapid heartbeat, and seizures. If you experience any of these symptoms, go to the nearest hospital emergency room immediately.

Pregnancy and Lactation

Bupropion should only be taken during pregnancy if the potential benefits clearly outweigh any potential risks to the fetus. If you are pregnant or plan to become pregnant, notify your doctor immediately.

The drug may pass into breast milk and may be harmful to a nursing infant. If the medication is essential to your health, your doctor may advise you not to breast-feed while you are taking it.

Buspirone

Brand Name
BuSpar

General Information
Buspirone is used to treat anxiety disorders. While its mechanism of action is unknown, it has complex interactions with the neurotransmitters dopamine and serotonin.

Symptoms of anxiety include trembling, twitching, heart palpitations, shortness of breath, sweaty palms, clammy skin, dry mouth, dizziness, nausea, and trouble swallowing.

Side Effects
More common side effects may include chest pain, dizziness, dream disturbances, headache, lightheadedness, nasal congestion, nausea, nervousness, ringing in the ears, sore throat, and unusual excitement.

Less common or rare side effects may include altered sense of taste or smell; conjunctivitis; changes in appetite; changes in sexual function; chest congestion; dry skin; easy bruising; exaggerated feeling of well-being; eye pain; fearfulness; fever; fluid retention; flushing; frequent or painful urination; gas; general loss of interest; hair loss; hallucinations; heart attack or heart failure; high or low blood pressure; intolerance of light; itching; joint pain; loss of sensation anywhere in the body; loss of strength or fainting; menstrual irregularities; muscle pain, spasms, or cramps; muscle weakness; pain or weakness in the hands or feet; rectal bleeding; red and itchy eyes; restlessness; seizures; shortness of breath; slow heartbeat; slurred speech; stroke; stupor; tingling sensation; uncontrolled body movements; and urinary incontinence.

If you experience any of these side effects or reactions, notify your doctor as soon as possible.

Important Precautions

Do not take buspirone if you have severe liver or kidney damage, if you are taking a type of antidepressant called a monoamine oxidase inhibitor (MAOI) or have taken one within the past two weeks, or if you have ever had an allergic reaction or hypersensitivity to buspirone or a similar drug.

Buspirone may make you feel dizzy and drowsy. Do not drive, operate machinery, or participate in any high-risk activities until you know exactly how the drug affects you.

Food and Drug Interactions

If buspirone is taken with certain other drugs, the effects of either drug could be increased, decreased, or changed. Before beginning treatment with buspirone, tell your doctor if you are taking any other prescription or over-the-counter medications.

Buspirone should not be combined with MAOIs. It is also important to check with your doctor before taking buspirone with haloperidol (Haldol) or trazodone (Desyrel).

Avoid drinking alcohol while taking buspirone.

Recommended Dosage

Usual dosage for adults: The usual starting dose is 15 mg a day taken in several divided doses, usually 5 mg three times a day. If necessary, this amount may gradually be increased by increments of 5 mg until an effective dose is reached. Dosages above 60 mg a day are not recommended.

Usual dosage for the elderly: 15 mg a day taken in several divided doses.

The safety and effectiveness of buspirone use in children under the age of eighteen has not been established.

Overdosage

Symptoms of a buspirone overdose may include drowsiness, nausea or vomiting, severe stomach upset, and pinpoint pupils. If you experience any of these symptoms, go to the nearest hospital emergency room immediately.

Pregnancy and Lactation

The safety of buspirone use during pregnancy has not been established. If you are pregnant or plan to become pregnant, notify your doctor immediately.

The drug may pass into breast milk and may be harmful to a nursing infant. If the medication is essential to your health, your doctor may advise you not to breast-feed while you are taking it.

Carbamazepine

Brand Names
Atretol, Tegretol

General Information

Carbamazepine is an anticonvulsant drug used to treat seizure disorders such as epilepsy. It is also sometimes prescribed for the treatment of bipolar or manic-depressive illness, although it has not been approved by the FDA for this purpose. Specifically, it helps to keep the manic phase of the condition under control. Carbamazepine may work via effects on the neurotransmitter GABA (gamma-aminobutyric acid).

Symptoms of mania include elation, hyperactivity, flight of ideas, rapid speech, grandiose ideas, hostility, decreased need for sleep, and uncharacteristically poor judgment.

Side Effects

Common side effects, experienced most often at the beginning of treatment, may include dizziness, drowsiness, nausea, unsteadiness, and vomiting.

The most serious side effects involve the blood, cardiovascular system, and skin. They may include abdominal pain; abnormal heartbeat; aching joints and muscles; acute skin inflammation; agitation; aplastic anemia; blood clots; blurred vision; chills; confusion; congestive heart failure; conjunctivitis; constipation; depression; diarrhea; double vision; dry mouth and throat; fainting; fatigue; fever; fluid retention; frequent urination; hair loss; hallucinations; headache; hepatitis; high blood pressure; hives; impotence; inflammation of the lungs; inflammation of the mouth and tongue; involuntary movements; kidney failure; labored breathing; leg cramps; liver disorders; loss of appetite; loss of coordination; low blood pressure; peeling skin; pneumonia; reddish or purplish spots on the skin; reduced urinary volume; ringing in the ears; sensitivity to light; skin pigmentation changes; skin rashes; speech difficulties; stomach problems; suppression of bone marrow's ability to make red and white blood cells; sweating; talkativeness; tingling sensation; and yellow eyes and skin.

If you experience any of these side effects or reactions, notify your doctor as soon as possible.

Important Precautions

Since carbamazepine can cause life-threatening adverse reactions such as aplastic anemia, bone marrow depression, and decreased white blood cell count, your complete blood count must be monitored regularly while you are taking the drug. Periodic evaluations of your liver and kidney function must also be performed throughout treatment.

Do not take carbamazepine if you have a history of bone marrow depression or if you have ever had an allergic reaction or sensitivity to carbamazepine, to tricyclic antidepressants, or to monoamine oxidase inhibitors. This drug may also not be appropriate for people with a history of heart, liver, or kidney dysfunction, glaucoma, or an adverse blood reaction to any drug. If you have suffered from any of these conditions, be sure to discuss the details thoroughly with your doctor before taking carbamazepine.

Carbamazepine may make you feel dizzy and drowsy. Do not drive, operate machinery, or participate in any high-risk activities until you know exactly how the drug affects you.

Abruptly discontinuing treatment with this medication can produce severe withdrawal symptoms.

Never take carbamazepine on an empty stomach.

Food and Drug Interactions

If carbamazepine is taken with certain other drugs, the effects of either drug could be increased, decreased, or changed. Before beginning treatment with carbamazepine, tell your doctor if you are taking any other prescription or over-the-counter medications.

Other anticonvulsant medications such as phenobarbital (Donnatal), phenytoin (Dilantin), and primidone (Mysoline) may decrease the effectiveness of carbamazepine.

Cimetidine (Tagamet), the antibiotic erythromycin, isoniazid (INH), propoxyphene (Darvon), and calcium channel blockers such as verapamil may cause carbamazepine to become toxic.

The effectiveness of the antibiotic doxycycline,

haloperidol (Haldol), phenytoin (Dilantin), theophylline (Theo-Dur), valproic acid (Depakene, Depakote), and warfarin (Coumadin) may be reduced when taken in conjunction with carbamazepine.

The use of lithium with carbamazepine may cause serious nervous system side effects.

The combination of carbamazepine and oral contraceptives may result in breakthrough bleeding. The reliability of the birth control pills may also be negatively affected.

Recommended Dosage

The recommended daily dose of carbamazepine depends upon the condition that is being treated.

Usual dosage for adults: 200 to 1,200 mg a day.

Usual dosage for children aged six to twelve: 200 to 1,000 mg a day.

Carbamazepine is not recommended for children under the age of six. It may cause confusion or agitation in elderly people.

Overdosage

The initial signs of a carbamazepine overdose usually surface within one to three hours. The most obvious symptoms include coma, convulsions, dizziness, drowsiness, irregular or reduced breathing, lack of coordination, lack of urine, low or high blood pressure, muscular twitching, nausea, pupil dilation, rapid eye movements, rapid heartbeat, restlessness, severe muscle spasms, shock, tremors, unconsciousness, and vomiting. If you experience any of these symptoms, go to the nearest hospital emergency room immediately.

Pregnancy and Lactation

Carbamazepine has been reported to cause birth defects such as spina bifida. For this reason, it should only be used during pregnancy if the potential benefit clearly outweighs the potential risk. If you are pregnant or plan to become pregnant, notify your doctor immediately.

The drug also passes into breast milk and may be harmful to a nursing infant. If the medication is essential to your health, your doctor may advise you not to breast-feed while you are taking it.

Chlordiazepoxide

Brand Names

Libritabs, Librium

General Information

Chlordiazepoxide is used in the treatment of anxiety disorders. It is also used to relieve the symptoms of alcohol withdrawal. It is a member of the class of drugs called benzodiazepines, which facilitate the action of the neurotransmitter GABA (gamma-aminobutyric acid). At lower doses, chlordiazepoxide decreases anxiety. At higher doses, it causes sedation and sleep. Chlordiazepoxide relaxes skeletal muscles as well.

Symptoms of anxiety include trembling, twitching, heart palpitations, shortness of breath, sweaty palms, clammy skin, dry mouth, dizziness, nausea, and trouble swallowing.

Side Effects

More common side effects may include confusion, drowsiness, and lack of muscle coordination.

Less common or rare side effects may include constipation; fainting; increased or decreased sex drive; minor menstrual irregularities; nausea; skin rash or eruptions; stiffness; swelling due to fluid retention; and yellowing of the skin and whites of the eyes.

If you experience any of these side effects or reactions, notify your doctor as soon as possible.

Important Precautions

Do not take chlordiazepoxide if you have ever had an allergic reaction or hypersensitivity to it or a similar drug.

Use this medication with caution if you are severely depressed or have a history of severe depression, or if you suffer from kidney or liver disease or a rare metabolic disorder called porphyria.

Chlordiazepoxide may make you drowsy or less alert. Do not drive, operate machinery, or participate in any high-risk activities until you know exactly how the drug affects you.

Abruptly discontinuing chlordiazepoxide may result in withdrawal symptoms such as abdominal and muscle cramps, convulsions, increase in the severity of anxiety symptoms, perspiration, tremors, and vomiting. When ending treatment with this medication, follow your doctor's schedule for a gradual withdrawal.

Food and Drug Interactions

If chlordiazepoxide is taken with certain other drugs, the effects of either drug could be increased, decreased, or changed. Before beginning treatment with chlordiazepoxide, tell your doctor if you are taking any other prescription or over-the-counter medications.

It is particularly important to check with your doctor before combining chlordiazepoxide with blood thinners, barbiturates, monoamine oxidase inhibitors, narcotics, and tranquilizers known as phenothiazines.

Do not drink alcohol while taking chlordiazepoxide.

Recommended Dosage

Usual dosage for adults: 5 or 10 mg three or four times a day for mild to moderate anxiety; 20 to 25 mg three or four times a day for severe anxiety.

Usual dosage for the elderly: 5 mg two to four times a day.

Usual dosage for children six years of age or older: 5 mg two to four times a day. If necessary, this amount may gradually be increased to 10 mg two or three times a day.

Chlordiazepoxide is not recommended for children under the age of six.

Overdosage

Symptoms of a chlordiazepoxide overdose may include coma, confusion, sleepiness, and slowed reflexes. If you experience any of these symptoms, go to the nearest hospital emergency room immediately.

Pregnancy and Lactation

Chlordiazepoxide may cause birth defects. As a result, it should not be taken during pregnancy. If you are pregnant or plan to become pregnant, notify your doctor immediately.

The drug may pass into breast milk and may be harmful to a nursing infant. If the medication is essential to your health, your doctor may advise you not to breast-feed while you are taking it.

Chlorpromazine

Brand Name
Thorazine

General Information

Chlorpromazine is used in the treatment of psychotic disorders such as schizophrenia. It works by blocking the neurotransmitter dopamine. This suggests that many of the symptoms of psychosis may result from abnormal dopamine activity in the brain.

Symptoms of schizophrenia include delusions, hallucinations, disorganized speech, grossly disorganized or catatonic behavior, and absence of normal moods and emotions.

Side Effects

Chlorpromazine may cause neuroleptic malignant syndrome (NMS), a rare but potentially life-threatening side effect characterized by severe muscle rigidity throughout the body. Other features of NMS include high fever, rapid heartbeat, rapid breathing, excessive perspiration, abnormal blood pressure, and kidney failure.

This drug also may cause a serious, and at times permanent, side effect called tardive dyskinesia. This neurological syndrome results in involuntary movements of the mouth, lips, and tongue such as tongue rolling, lip licking and smacking, chewing or sucking motions, pouting, and grimacing.

Other side effects may include abnormal secretion of milk; abnormal sugar in urine; agitation; anemia; asthma; blood disorders; breast development in males; chewing movements; constipation; difficulty breathing; difficulty swallowing; drooling; drowsiness; ejaculation problems; fever; fixed gaze; fluid retention and swelling; flulike symptoms; headache; heart attack; high or low blood sugar; hives; impotence; infections; intestinal blockage; involuntary movements of the arms, legs, tongue, face, mouth, or jaw; irregular blood pressure, pulse, and heartbeat; irregular or absence of menstrual periods; masklike facial expression; muscle stiffness and rigidity; narrow or dilated pupils; nasal congestion; nausea; nervousness; pain and stiffness in the neck; persistent, painful erections; protruding tongue; puckering of the mouth; puffing of the cheeks; rigid arms, feet, head, and muscles; seizures; sensitivity to light; severe allergic reactions; shuffling gait; sore throat; spasms in the jaw, face, tongue, neck, mouth, and feet; sweating; swelling of breasts; tremors; twitching in the body, neck, shoulders, and face; and visual problems.

Less common or rare side effects may include abnormalities in movement and posture; dizziness; dry mouth; fainting; increase of appetite; insomnia; lightheadedness upon standing up; rapid heartbeat; skin inflammation and peeling; weight gain; and yellowing of the skin and whites of the eyes.

If you experience any of these side effects or reactions, notify your doctor as soon as possible.

Important Precautions

Keep in mind that chlorpromazine can cause neuroleptic malignant syndrome and tardive dyskinesia.

Do not take chlorpromazine if you are also taking central nervous system depressants.

Use this medication with caution if you have ever had asthma; a brain tumor; breast cancer; emphysema; glaucoma; heart, kidney, or liver disease; intestinal blockage; seizures; or a bone marrow or blood disorder. Chlorpromazine should also be used cautiously by people who are exposed to extreme heat or pesticides.

Chlorpromazine can mask the symptoms of brain tumors, intestinal blockage, and Reye's syndrome. Because it prevents vomiting, it can also mask the signs of an overdose of another drug. This medication can suppress the cough reflex as well. If you develop a fever or sore throat, mouth, or gums while taking chlorpromazine, inform your doctor immediately. These symptoms may indicate that you need to discontinue therapy.

Periodic evaluations of your blood, liver, and kidneys should be performed throughout treatment.

Chlorpromazine may make you drowsy and impair your coordination. Do not drive, operate machinery, or participate in any high-risk activities until you know exactly how the drug affects you.

Since chlorpromazine can make you sensitive to light, try to stay out of the sun as much as possible while taking it.

Abruptly discontinuing chlorpromazine may result in dizziness, nausea, stomach inflammation, tremors, and vomiting. When ending treatment with this medication, follow your doctor's schedule for a gradual withdrawal.

Food and Drug Interactions

If chlorpromazine is taken with certain other drugs, the effects of either drug could be increased, decreased, or changed. Before beginning treatment with chlorpromazine, tell your doctor if you are taking any other prescription or over-the-counter medications.

It is particularly important to check with your doctor before taking chlorpromazine with anesthetics, antacids, anticoagulants, anticonvulsants, barbiturates, diuretics, atropine (Donnatal), cimetidine (Tagamet), guanethidine (Ismelin), or propranolol (Inderal).

Chlorpromazine should not be combined with alcohol, narcotics, sleeping pills, or tranquilizers.

Recommended Dosage

Usual dosage for adults: The usual starting dose ranges from 30 to 75 mg a day taken in three or four divided doses. If necessary, this amount may gradually be increased by increments of 20 to 50 mg until an effective dose is reached.

Elderly people usually take lower doses of chlorpromazine since they have a higher risk of developing tardive dyskinesia and low blood pressure.

Dosages for children should be individually tailored by a doctor.

Overdosage

Symptoms of a chlorpromazine overdose may include agitation, coma, convulsions, difficulty breathing, difficulty swallowing, dry mouth, extreme sleepiness, fever, intestinal blockage, irregular heartbeat, and restlessness. If you experience any of these symptoms, go to the nearest hospital emergency room immediately.

Pregnancy and Lactation

Chlorpromazine should only be used during pregnancy if the potential benefits clearly outweigh any potential risks to the fetus. If you are pregnant or plan to become pregnant, notify your doctor immediately.

The drug passes into breast milk and may be harmful to a nursing infant. If the medication is essential to your health, your doctor may advise you not to breast-feed while you are taking it.

Clomipramine

Brand Name
Anafranil

General Information

Clomipramine is a tricyclic antidepressant used in the treatment of obsessive-compulsive disorder. It works by blocking the presynaptic reuptake of the neurotransmitters serotonin, norepinephrine, and dopamine in the brain. This suggests that many of the symptoms of depression may result from imbalances of one or more of these neurotransmitters.

Obsessions are intrusive, unwanted ideas, images, impulses, or worries that dominate a person's thoughts, such as fearing contamination or doubting whether the front door is locked. Compulsions are senseless, irrational rituals that a person feels driven to perform again and again, such as washing hands or checking the front door dozens of times a day.

Side Effects

Clomipramine is associated with an increased risk of seizures. Men who take this drug may become impotent or be unable to ejaculate. Many users of the medication experience unwanted weight gain. A small percentage, however, actually lose weight.

More common side effects may include confusion, drowsiness, nausea, and vomiting.

Other side effects may include abnormal thinking; abnormality in walking; acne; agitation; anxiety; back pain; changes in sex drive; chest pain; chills; confusion; constipation; cough; depression; diarrhea; difficulty breathing; difficulty urinating; dizziness; double vision; dream abnormalities; drowsiness; dry mouth; dry skin; earache; eye pain; fatigue; feelings of unreality; fever; gas; genital itching; headache; hives; hot flushes; impotence; increased appetite; increased perspiration; indecisiveness; insomnia; irritability; itching; loss of appetite; memory problems; menstrual pain and disorders; muscle jerks and twitching; nausea; nervousness; numbness; rapid heartbeat; rash; refusal or inability to speak; ringing in the ears; runny nose; sleep disturbances; sore throat; speech disturbances; stomach pain and upset; suicidal thoughts; taste changes; teeth grinding; tingling; tremors; urinary problems; vertigo; vision problems; vomiting; weakness; and yawning.

If you experience any of these side effects or reactions, notify your doctor as soon as possible.

Important Precautions

Do not take clomipramine if you are recovering from a heart attack, if you are taking a type of antidepressant called a monoamine oxidase inhibitor (MAOI) or have taken one within the past two weeks, or if you have ever had an allergic reaction or hypersensitivity to a tricyclic antidepressant.

Use this medication with caution if you have a history of narrow-angle glaucoma or increased pressure in the eyes, urinary retention, or abnormal kidney function.

Your risk of experiencing seizures while taking clomipramine is increased if you have ever had a seizure in the past, if you have a history of brain damage or alcoholism, or if you are taking any other medications that might cause seizures.

If you have a tumor of the adrenal medulla, clomipramine could trigger a sudden, dangerous rise in blood pressure.

Clomipramine may make you feel dizzy and drowsy. Do not drive, operate machinery, or participate in any high-risk activities until you know exactly how the drug affects you.

Be sure to inform your doctor or dentist that you are taking clomipramine before undergoing any type of surgery or dental treatment requiring general anesthesia.

Since clomipramine can make you sensitive to light, try to stay out of the sun as much as possible during your treatment.

To avoid stomach upset, take clomipramine with food.

Abruptly discontinuing clomipramine may result in dizziness, fever, headaches, irritability, malaise, nausea, sleep problems, vomiting, and worsening of emotional or mental problems. When ending treatment with this medication, follow your doctor's schedule for a gradual withdrawal.

Food and Drug Interactions

If clomipramine is taken with certain other drugs, the effects of either drug could be increased, decreased, or changed. Before beginning treatment with clomipramine, tell your doctor if you are taking any other prescription or over-the-counter medications.

Combining clomipramine with a MAOI can lead to extremely high fever, severe convulsions, even death. If you have been taking a MAOI, you must wait at least two weeks after discontinuing therapy with the drug before starting therapy with clomipramine.

It is also important to check with your doctor before combining clomipramine with anticholinergic drugs such as Artane or Cogentin, antihypertensive drugs, psychoactive drugs, thyroid medications, cimetidine (Tagamet), digoxin (Lanoxin), fluoxetine (Prozac), haloperidol (Haldol), methylphenidate (Ritalin), or warfarin (Coumadin).

Do not drink alcohol while taking clomipramine.

Recommended Dosage

Usual dosage for adults: The usual starting dose is 25 mg a day. If necessary, this amount may gradually be increased to 100 mg a day during the first two weeks of treatment. Dosages above 200 mg a day are not recommended.

Usual dosage for children: The usual starting dose is 25 mg a day. If necessary, this amount may gradually be increased to a maximum of 100 mg a day or 3 mg per 2.2 pounds of body weight, whichever is smaller.

Overdosage

An overdose of clomipramine can be fatal. Early symptoms of overdose may include agitation, coma, convulsions, delirium, drowsiness, grimacing, hyperactive reflexes, loss of coordination, perspiration, restlessness, rigid muscles, staggering gait, stupor, and writhing. Other symptoms may include bluish skin, dilated pupils, fever, low blood pressure, shallow breathing, shock, vomiting, and urinary retention. A clomipramine overdose may also result in heart malfunction and even cardiac arrest in rare instances. If you experience any of these symptoms, go to the nearest hospital emergency room immediately.

Pregnancy and Lactation

Clomipramine should only be used during pregnancy if the potential benefits clearly outweigh any potential risks to the fetus. If you are pregnant or plan to become pregnant, notify your doctor immediately.

The drug passes into breast milk and may be harmful to a nursing infant. If the medication is essential to your health, your doctor may advise you not to breast-feed while you are taking it.

Clonazepam

Brand Name
Klonopin

General Information

Clonazepam is an anticonvulsant drug used in the treatment of seizure disorders. It may also be used in the short-term treatment of anxiety disorder and panic disorder, although it has not been approved by the FDA for this purpose. It is a member of the class of drugs called benzodiazepines, which facilitate the action of the neurotransmitter GABA (gamma-aminobutyric acid). At lower doses, clonazepam decreases anxiety. At higher doses, it causes sedation and sleep. Clonazepam relaxes skeletal muscles as well.

Symptoms of anxiety include trembling, twitching, heart palpitations, shortness of breath, sweaty palms, clammy skin, dry mouth, dizziness, nausea, and trouble swallowing.

Side Effects

More common side effects may include behavior problems (particularly in children), drowsiness, and lack of muscular coordination.

Less common or rare side effects may include anemia; chest congestion; coated tongue; confusion; constipation; depression; diarrhea; double vision; dry mouth; fecal incontinence; fever; fluid retention; glassy eyes; hair loss; hallucinations; involuntary rapid eye movement; loss of or increased appetite; loss of voice; memory loss; muscle weakness; nausea; painful or difficult urination; rapid heartbeat; rash; runny nose; shortness of breath; sore gums; speech difficulties; uncontrolled body movements; unusual bleeding or bruising; urinary incontinence; vertigo; and weight gain or loss.

If you experience any of these side effects or reactions, notify your doctor as soon as possible.

Important Precautions

Do not take clonazepam if you have acute narrow-angle glaucoma or severe liver disease, or if you have ever had an allergic reaction or hypersensitivity to clonazepam or a similar drug.

Ambien

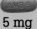

5 mg

10 mg

Anafranil

25 mg

50 mg

Asendin

50 mg

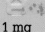

100 mg

Ativan

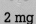

1 mg

2 mg

BuSpar

5 mg

10 mg

Clozaril

25 mg

100 mg

Cognex

10 mg

30 mg

Cylert

18.75 mg

37.5 mg

Dalmane

15 mg

30 mg

Depakote

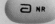

250 mg

500 mg

Desyrel

50 mg

100 mg

Dexedrine

5 mg

10 mg

Doral

7.5 mg

Effexor

37.5 mg

100 mg

Elavil

25 mg

50 mg

Eskalith

300 mg

450 mg

Halcion

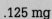

.125 mg

.25 mg

Haldol

10 mg

20 mg

Klonopin

1 mg

2 mg

Librium

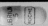

5 mg

10 mg

Loxitane

25 mg

50 mg

Ludiomil

25 mg

50 mg

Moban

25 mg

50 mg

Nardil

15 mg

Luvox

50 mg

100 mg

Navane

10 mg

20 mg

Mellaril

25 mg

100 mg

Norpramin

50 mg

150 mg

Orap

2 mg

ProSom

1 mg

2 mg

Pamelor

50 mg

75 mg

Parnate

10 mg

Prozac

10 mg

20 mg

Paxil

20 mg

30 mg

Restoril

15 mg

30 mg

Risperdal

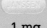

1 mg

3 mg

Ritalin

5 mg

10 mg

20 mg

Serax

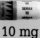

10 mg

15 mg

Serentil

50 mg

100 mg

Serzone

100 mg

200 mg

Sinequan

25 mg

150 mg

Stelazine

2 mg

10 mg

Thorazine

50 mg

100 mg

Surmontil

50 mg

100 mg

Tofranil

25 mg

50 mg

Tegretol

100 mg

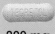

200 mg

Tranxene

3.75 mg

7.5 mg

Trilafon

2 mg

16 mg

Wellbutrin

75 mg

100 mg

Valium

5 mg

Xanax

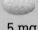

.5 mg

1 mg

Vivactil

5 mg

10 mg

Zoloft

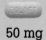

50 mg

100 mg

Use this medication with caution if you suffer from several different types of seizure disorders since it may increase the possibility of experiencing grand mal seizures.

Clonazepam may make you drowsy or less alert. Do not drive, operate machinery, or participate in any high-risk activities until you know exactly how the drug affects you.

Abruptly discontinuing clonazepam may result in withdrawal symptoms such as abdominal and muscle cramps, behavior disorders, convulsions, hallucination, psychosis, restlessness, sleeping difficulties, and tremors. When ending treatment with this medication, follow your doctor's schedule for a gradual withdrawal.

After many years of use, clonazepam may adversely affect a person's physical or mental development. Consequently, you and your doctor should carefully weigh the potential benefits of the drug against the potential risks.

Food and Drug Interactions

If clonazepam is taken with certain other drugs, the effects of either drug could be increased, decreased, or changed. Before beginning treatment with clonazepam, tell your doctor if you are taking any other prescription or over-the-counter medications.

It is particularly important to check with your doctor before combining clonazepam with other antianxiety agents, other anticonvulsants, antipsychotic drugs, barbiturates, hypnotic drugs, monoamine oxidase inhibitors, narcotics, tricyclic antidepressants, or valproic acid (Depakene, Depakote).

Do not drink alcohol while taking clonazepam.

Recommended Dosage

Usual dosage for adults: The starting dose should not exceed 1.5 mg a day taken in three divided doses. If necessary, this amount may gradually be increased until an effective dose is reached. Dosages above 20 mg a day are not recommended.

Usual dosage for children: The starting dose for children up to ten years of age or up to sixty-six pounds should be between .01 and .03 mg per 2.2 pounds of body weight taken each day in two or three divided doses. If necessary, this amount may gradually be increased until an effective dose is reached.

Overdosage

Symptoms of a clonazepam overdose may include coma, confusion, sleepiness, and slowed reflexes. If you experience any of these symptoms, go to the nearest hospital emergency room immediately.

Pregnancy and Lactation

The safety of clonazepam use during pregnancy has not been established. If you are pregnant or plan to become pregnant, notify your doctor immediately.

The drug may pass into breast milk and may be harmful to a nursing infant. If the medication is essential to your health, your doctor may advise you not to breast-feed while you are taking it.

Clorazepate

Brand Name

Tranxene

General Information

Clorazepate is used in the treatment of anxiety disorders. It is a member of the class of drugs called benzodiazepines, which facilitate the action of the neurotransmitter GABA (gamma-aminobutyric acid). At lower doses, clorazepate decreases anxiety. At higher doses, it causes sedation and sleep. Clorazepate relaxes skeletal muscles as well.

Symptoms of anxiety include trembling, twitching, heart palpitations, shortness of breath, sweaty palms, clammy skin, dry mouth, dizziness, nausea, and trouble swallowing.

Other conditions clorazepate may be prescribed for include alcohol withdrawal, anxiety associated with depression, and convulsive disorders such as epilepsy.

Side Effects

More common side effects may include drowsiness.

Less common or rare side effects may include blurred vision; confusion; depression; dizziness; double vision; dry mouth; fatigue; genital and urinary tract disorders; headache; insomnia; irritability; lack of muscle coordination; nervousness; rash; slurred speech; stomach and intestinal disorders; and tremors.

If you experience any of these side effects or reactions, notify your doctor as soon as possible.

Important Precautions

Do not take clorazepate if you have acute narrow-angle glaucoma or if you have ever had an allergic reaction or hypersensitivity to clorazepate or a similar drug.

Clorazepate may make you drowsy or less alert. Do not drive, operate machinery, or participate in any high-risk activities until you know exactly how the drug affects you.

Abruptly discontinuing clorazepate may result in withdrawal symptoms such as diarrhea, hallucinations, impaired memory, insomnia, irritability, muscle aches, nervousness, and tremors. When ending treatment with this medication, follow your doctor's schedule for a gradual withdrawal.

Food and Drug Interactions

If clorazepate is taken with certain other drugs, the effects of either drug could be increased, decreased, or changed. Before beginning treatment with clorazepate, tell your doctor if you are taking any other prescription or over-the-counter medications.

It is particularly important to check with your doctor before combining clorazepate with antidepressant drugs called monoamine oxidase inhibitors, any other antidepressants, barbiturates, narcotics, and tranquilizers known as phenothiazines.

Do not drink alcohol while taking clorazepate.

Recommended Dosage

Usual dosage for adults: 30 mg a day taken in several divided doses. If necessary, this amount may gradually be increased to a maximum of 60 mg a day.

Some people require as little as 15 mg a day. Clorazepate is also available in a single bedtime dose; a 22.5-mg tablet that can be taken once a day; and an 11.25-mg tablet that can be taken once a day.

Usual dosage for the elderly: The usual starting dose is 7.5 to 15 mg a day.

Clorazepate may be used in conjunction with anti-convulsant drugs in children nine years of age and older. The safety and effectiveness of clorazepate use in children under the age of nine has not been established.

Overdosage

Symptoms of a clorazepate overdose may include coma, low blood pressure, and sedation. If you experience any of these symptoms, go to the nearest hospital emergency room immediately.

Pregnancy and Lactation

Clorazepate may cause birth defects. As a result, it should not be taken during pregnancy. If you are pregnant or plan to become pregnant, notify your doctor immediately.

The drug may pass into breast milk and may be harmful to a nursing infant. If the medication is essential to your health, your doctor may advise you not to breast-feed while you are taking it.

Clozapine

Brand Name
Clozaril

General Information

Clozapine is an antipsychotic drug used in the treatment of severe schizophrenia that has not responded to standard antipsychotic medications. It works by blocking the neurotransmitters dopamine and serotonin. Clozapine also binds strongly to the recently described class of dopamine receptors called D4 receptors. These facts suggest that some of the symptoms of psychosis may result from abnormal dopamine and serotonin activity in the brain.

Symptoms of schizophrenia include delusions, hallucinations, disorganized speech, grossly disorganized or catatonic behavior, and absence of normal moods and emotions.

Side Effects

Clozapine may cause a potentially fatal disorder of the white blood cells called agranulocytosis. For this reason, the drug is prescribed only to individuals who comply with mandatory weekly blood tests. Approximately 1 percent of users develop the condition and must stop taking the medication.

Another potential side effect is seizures, which occur in approximately 5 percent of people who take clozapine, particularly those on high doses.

More common side effects may include constipation; dizziness; drowsiness; dry mouth; fainting; fever; low blood pressure; nausea; rapid heartbeat and other heart conditions; salivation; sedation; sweating; tremors; vertigo; vision problems; and vomiting.

Less common side effects may include abnormal stools; backache; bitter taste; bloodshot eyes; breast pain or discomfort; bruising; chills; confusion; coughing; dry throat; ear disorders; ejaculation problems; hallucinations; headache; hives; hot flashes; impotence; increase in appetite; increase or decrease in sex drive; involuntary movement of the eyes; irritability; itching; joint pain; lethargy; light-headedness; loss of speech; muscle pain; nervous stomach; nosebleed; numbness; pneumonia-like symptoms; poor coordination; pounding heartbeat; rash; rectal bleeding; restlessness; runny nose; shakiness; skin inflammation; sleeplessness; sneezing; sore throat; stomach pain; stuttering; twitching; vaginal itch; vague feeling of being sick; weakness; and wheezing.

If you experience any of these side effects or reactions, notify your doctor as soon as possible.

Important Precautions

Keep in mind that clozapine can cause agranulocytosis and seizures.

Do not take clozapine if you have ever had a bone-marrow disease or disorder, if you are taking another drug that might cause a decrease in white blood cell count, or if you have ever developed an abnormally low white blood cell count while taking clozapine.

Use this medication with caution if you have a history of heart, kidney, or liver disease, low blood pressure, narrow-angle glaucoma, prostate problems, or seizures. If you have suffered from any of these conditions, be sure to discuss the details thoroughly with your doctor before taking clozapine.

Clozapine may make you feel drowsy. Do not drive, operate machinery, or participate in any high-risk activities until you know exactly how the drug affects you.

Although your blood will be tested on a weekly basis during clozapine therapy, it is important to monitor yourself for the early warning signs of agranulocytosis—canker sores in the mouth, fever, flulike feeling, lethargy, malaise, sore throat, and weakness. If you develop any of these symptoms, inform your doctor immediately.

Food and Drug Interactions

If clozapine is taken with certain other drugs, the effects of either drug could be increased, decreased, or changed. Before beginning treatment with clozapine, tell your doctor if you are taking any other prescription or over-the-counter medications.

It is particularly important to check with your doctor before taking clozapine with blood pressure medications, central nervous system depressants, drugs that contain atropine (such as Donnatal and Lomotil), drugs that suppress bone-marrow activity (such as carbamazepine), digoxin (Lanoxin), or warfarin (Coumadin).

Throughout treatment with clozapine, do not drink alcoholic beverages or take drugs of any kind, including over-the-counter medications, before consulting with your doctor.

Recommended Dosage

Usual dosage for adults: The usual starting dose is 25 mg once or twice a day. If necessary, this amount may gradually be increased by increments of 25 to 50 mg a day until a daily dose of 300 to 450 mg is reached. Dosages above 900 mg are not recommended due to increased risk of seizures.

The safety and effectiveness of clozapine in children under the age of sixteen has not been established.

Overdosage

Symptoms of a clozapine overdose may include coma, delirium, drowsiness, excessive salivation, faintness, low blood pressure, rapid heartbeat, seizures, and shallow breathing. If you experience any of these symptoms, go to the nearest hospital emergency room immediately.

Pregnancy and Lactation

The safety of clozapine use during pregnancy has not been established. If you are pregnant or plan to become pregnant, notify your doctor immediately.

The drug may pass into breast milk and may be harmful to a nursing infant. If the medication is essential to your health, your doctor may advise you not to breast-feed while you are taking it.

Desipramine

Brand Name
Norpramin

General Information
Desipramine is used in the treatment of depression. It is a member of the class of drugs called tricyclic antidepressants, which work by blocking the presynaptic reuptake of the neurotransmitters serotonin, norepinephrine, and dopamine in the brain. This suggests that many of the symptoms of depression may result from imbalances of one or more of these neurotransmitters.

Symptoms of depression include low, anxious, or "empty" feelings; loss of interest and pleasure in activities previously enjoyed; noticeable change of appetite; noticeable change in sleeping patterns; fatigue or loss of energy; feelings of hopelessness or pessimism; feelings of guilt, worthlessness, or helplessness; inability to concentrate, make decisions, or remember details; recurring thoughts of death or suicide, wishing to die or attempting suicide; and aches and pains, constipation, or other physical ailments that cannot be explained.

Side Effects
Side effects may include abdominal cramps; agitation; anxiety; black, red, or blue spots on the skin; black tongue; blurred vision; breast development in males; confusion; constipation; delusions; diarrhea; dilated pupils; disorientation; dizziness; drowsiness;

dry mouth; excessive or spontaneous flow of milk; fatigue; fever; flushing; frequent urination or difficulty or delay in urinating; hair loss; hallucinations; headache; heart attack; hepatitis; high blood pressure; high or low blood sugar; hives; impotence; increased or decreased sex drive; inflammation of the mouth; insomnia; intestinal blockage; lack of coordination; light-headedness; loss of appetite; nausea; nightmares; odd taste in mouth; painful ejaculation; palpitations; restlessness; ringing in the ears; seizures; sensitivity to light; skin itching and rash; sore throat; stomach pain; stroke; sweating; swelling in the face or tongue; swelling of the breasts or testicles; swollen glands; tingling and numbness in the hands and feet; tremors; urinating at night; visual problems; vomiting; weakness; weight gain or loss; and yellowed skin and whites of eyes.

If you experience any of these side effects or reactions, notify your doctor as soon as possible.

Important Precautions

Do not take desipramine if you are recovering from a heart attack, if you are taking a type of antidepressant called a monoamine oxidase inhibitor (MAOI), or if you have ever had an allergic reaction or hypersensitivity to desipramine or a similar drug.

Use this medication with caution if you have a history of heart or thyroid disease, seizures, or urinary retention.

Desipramine may make you feel dizzy and drowsy. Do not drive, operate machinery, or participate in any high-risk activities until you know exactly how the drug affects you.

If you develop a sore throat or fever while taking desipramine, be sure to inform your doctor.

Abruptly discontinuing desipramine may result in headaches, nausea, and malaise. When ending treatment with this medication, follow your doctor's schedule for a gradual withdrawal.

Food and Drug Interactions

If desipramine is taken with certain other drugs, the effects of either drug could be increased, decreased, or changed. Before beginning treatment with desipramine, tell your doctor if you are taking any other prescription or over-the-counter medications.

Desipramine should not be combined with MAOIs. It is also important to check with your doctor before taking desipramine with sedative or hypnotic drugs, muscle relaxants, thyroid medications, albuterol (Proventil, Ventolin), cimetidine (Tagamet), fluoxetine (Prozac), or guanethidine (Ismelin).

Desipramine should not be taken with alcohol, sleeping pills, tranquilizers, or narcotic painkillers.

Recommended Dosage

Usual dosage for adults: 100 to 200 mg a day.
Usual dosage for adolescents and the elderly: 25 to 100 mg a day.
Desipramine is not recommended for children.

Overdosage

An overdose of desipramine can be fatal. Symptoms of overdose may include agitation, bluish or yellowish skin, coma, extremely low blood pressure, fever, irregular heart rate, kidney failure, palpitations, rigid muscles, seizures, shock, stupor, and vomiting. If you experience any of these symptoms, go to the nearest hospital emergency room immediately.

Pregnancy and Lactation

Desipramine should only be used during pregnancy if the potential benefits clearly outweigh any potential risks to the fetus. If you are pregnant or plan to become pregnant, notify your doctor immediately.

Similarly, the drug should only be used by a nursing mother if the potential benefits of therapy clearly outweigh any potential risks to the infant.

Dextroamphetamine

Brand Name

Dexedrine

General Information

Dextroamphetamine is a central nervous system stimulant used in the treatment of attention deficit disorder. It appears to work via effects on the neurotransmitter dopamine and/or the neurotransmitter norepinephrine.

Symptoms of attention deficit disorder include a chronic history of extreme distractibility, short attention span, physical or cognitive restlessness, impulsiveness, low tolerance for frustration, and mood swings.

This drug is also used to treat narcolepsy, a neurological condition characterized by an uncontrollable desire to sleep.

Side Effects

More common side effects may include excessive restlessness or overstimulation.

Other side effects may include altered sexual desire; appetite suppression; constipation; diarrhea; dizziness; dry mouth; euphoria; headache; heart palpitations; high blood pressure; hives; impotence; insomnia; rapid heartbeat; stomach and intestinal disturbances; tremors; uncontrollable twitching or jerking; unpleasant taste in the mouth; and weight loss.

If you experience any of these side effects or reactions, notify your doctor as soon as possible.

Important Precautions

Do not take dextroamphetamine if you suffer from agitation, cardiovascular disease, glaucoma, hardening of the arteries, high blood pressure, or thyroid overactivity; if you are taking a type of antidepressant called a monoamine oxidase inhibitor (MAOI) or have taken one within the past two weeks; if you have a history of alcohol or drug abuse; or if you have ever had an allergic reaction or hypersensitivity to dextroamphetamine or a similar drug.

Dextroamphetamine may make you feel dizzy and impair your coordination. Do not drive, operate machinery, or participate in any high-risk activities until you know exactly how the drug affects you.

Children should be carefully monitored during

treatment with dextroamphetamine since the drug may suppress growth.

Taking this drug late in the day can cause insomnia.

Some people, especially those who are allergic to aspirin, have experienced a severe allergic reaction to the yellow food coloring contained in dextroamphetamine.

Food and Drug Interactions

If dextroamphetamine is taken with certain other drugs, the effects of either drug could be increased, decreased, or changed. Before beginning treatment with dextroamphetamine, tell your doctor if you are taking any other prescription or over-the-counter medications.

Combining dextroamphetamine with a MAOI can lead to a sudden, potentially life-threatening rise in blood pressure. If you have been taking a MAOI, you must wait at least two weeks after discontinuing therapy with the drug before starting therapy with dextroamphetamine.

Substances that lessen the effects of dextroamphetamine include chlorpromazine (Thorazine), fruit juices, glutamic acid hydrochloride, guanethidine (Ismelin), haloperidol (Haldol), lithium (Eskalith, Lithobid), methenamine (Urised), reserpine (Serpasil), and vitamin C.

Substances that enhance the effects of dextroamphetamine include acetazolamide (Diamox), baking soda, diuretics, MAOIs, and propoxyphene hydrochloride (Darvon).

Substances that have decreased effect when taken with dextroamphetamine include adrenergic blockers such as propranolol (Inderal), antihistamines, blood pressure medications, and ethosuximide (Zarontin).

Substances that have increased effect when taken with dextroamphetamine include meperidine hydrochloride (Demerol), norepinephrine (Levophed), phenobarbital, phenytoin (Dilantin), and tricyclic antidepressants.

Recommended Dosage

The recommended daily dosage of dextroamphetamine depends upon whether it is being used to treat attention deficit disorder or narcolepsy.

Narcolepsy

Usual dosage for adults: 5 to 60 mg a day taken in several divided doses.

Usual dosage for children aged six to twelve: The usual starting dose is 5 mg a day. If necessary, this amount may gradually be increased by 5-mg increments until an effective dosage is reached.

Usual dosage for children aged twelve and older: The usual starting dose is 10 mg a day. This amount may gradually be increased by 10-mg increments until an effective dosage is reached.

Attention Deficit Disorder

Usual dosage for adults: 30 to 60 mg a day taken in several divided doses.

Usual dosage for children aged three to five: The usual starting dose is 2.5 mg a day, in tablet or elixir form. If necessary, this amount may gradually be increased by 2.5-mg increments until an effective dosage is reached.

Usual dosage for children aged six and older: The usual starting dose is 5 mg taken once or twice a day. If necessary, this amount may gradually be increased by 5-mg increments until an effective dosage is reached. Dosages above 40 mg are generally not recommended.

Sustained-release capsules, which can be taken once a day, are also available.

The safety and effectiveness of dextroamphetamine use in children under the age of three has not been established.

Overdosage

Symptoms of a severe dextroamphetamine overdose may include abdominal cramps; coma; confusion; convulsions; diarrhea; fever; hallucinations; heightened reflexes; high or low blood pressure; irregular heartbeat; nausea; panic; rapid breathing; restlessness; tremors; and vomiting. If you experience any of these symptoms, go to the nearest hospital emergency room immediately.

Pregnancy and Lactation

Research suggests that dextroamphetamine may cause birth defects. As a result, it should only be taken during pregnancy if the potential benefits clearly outweigh any potential risks to the fetus. If you are pregnant or plan to become pregnant, notify your doctor immediately.

The drug passes into breast milk and may be harmful to a nursing infant. If the medication is essential to your health, your doctor may advise you not to breast-feed while you are taking it.

Diazepam

Brand Name

Valium

General Information

Diazepam is used in the treatment of anxiety disorders. It is a member of the class of drugs called benzodiazepines, which facilitate the action of the neurotransmitter GABA (gamma-aminobutyric acid). At lower doses, diazepam decreases anxiety. At higher doses, it causes sedation and sleep. Diazepam relaxes skeletal muscles as well.

Symptoms of anxiety include trembling, twitching, heart palpitations, shortness of breath, sweaty palms, clammy skin, dry mouth, dizziness, nausea, and trouble swallowing.

Diazepam may also be prescribed for alcohol withdrawal and convulsive disorders such as epilepsy.

Side Effects

More common side effects may include drowsiness, light-headedness, loss of muscle coordination, and mild fatigue.

Less common or rare side effects may include anxiety; blurred vision; changes in salivation; changes in sex drive; confusion; constipation; depression; dizziness; double vision; hallucinations; headache; incontinence; low blood pressure; nausea; overexcitation; rash; seizures; sleep disturbances; slow heartbeat; slurred speech; tremors; urinary retention; and yellowing of the skin and whites of the eyes.

If you experience any of these side effects or reactions, notify your doctor as soon as possible.

Important Precautions

Do not take diazepam if you have acute narrow-angle glaucoma, if you are being treated for a mental illness more severe than anxiety, or if you have ever had an allergic reaction or hypersensitivity to diazepam or a similar drug.

Diazepam may make you drowsy or less alert. Do not drive, operate machinery, or participate in any high-risk activities until you know exactly how the drug affects you.

Abruptly discontinuing diazepam may result in withdrawal symptoms such as abdominal and muscle cramps, convulsions, perspiration, tremors, and vomiting. When ending treatment with this medication, follow your doctor's schedule for a gradual withdrawal.

Food and Drug Interactions

If diazepam is taken with certain other drugs, the effects of either drug could be increased, decreased, or changed. Before beginning treatment with diazepam, tell your doctor if you are taking any other prescription or over-the-counter medications.

It is particularly important to check with your doctor before combining diazepam with anticonvulsants, barbiturates, monoamine oxidase inhibitors, narcotics, oral contraceptives, cimetidine (Tagamet), disulfiram, fluoxetine (Prozac), isoniazid, levodopa (Larodopa), propoxyphene (Darvon), ranitidine (Zantac), and rifampin (Rifadin).

Do not drink alcohol while taking diazepam.

Recommended Dosage

Usual dosage for adults: 2 to 10 mg two to four times a day.

Usual dosage for the elderly: 2 to 2.5 mg one or two times a day.

Usual dosage for children: The usual starting dose for children over six months of age is 1 to 2.5 mg three or four times a day. This amount may gradually be increased.

Diazepam should not be used by children under six months of age.

Overdosage

Symptoms of a diazepam overdose may include coma, confusion, sleepiness, and slowed reflexes. If you experience any of these symptoms, go to the nearest hospital emergency room immediately.

Pregnancy and Lactation

Diazepam may cause birth defects. As a result, it should not be taken during pregnancy. If you are pregnant or plan to become pregnant, notify your doctor immediately.

The drug may pass into breast milk and may be harmful to a nursing infant. If the medication is essential to your health, your doctor may advise you not to breast-feed while you are taking it.

Doxepin

Brand Names

Adapin, Sinequan

General Information

Doxepin is used in the treatment of depression. It is a member of the class of drugs called tricyclic antidepressants, which work by blocking the presynaptic reuptake of the neurotransmitters serotonin, norepinephrine, and dopamine in the brain. This suggests that many of the symptoms of depression may result from imbalances of one or more of these neurotransmitters.

Symptoms of depression include low, anxious, or "empty" feelings; loss of interest and pleasure in activities previously enjoyed; noticeable change of appetite; noticeable change in sleeping patterns; fatigue or loss of energy; feelings of hopelessness or pessimism; feelings of guilt, worthlessness, or helplessness; inability to concentrate, make decisions, or remember details; recurring thoughts of death or suicide, wishing to die or attempting suicide; and aches and pains, constipation, or other physical ailments that cannot be explained.

Side Effects

A common side effect is drowsiness.

Less common or rare side effects may include blurred vision; breast development in males; breast enlargement; buzzing or ringing in the ears; chills; confusion; constipation; diarrhea; difficult urination;

disorientation; dizziness; dry mouth; excessive or spontaneous flow of milk; eye pain; fatigue; fluid retention; flushing; fragmented or incomplete movements; hair loss; hallucinations; headache; high fever; high or low blood sugar; increased or decreased sex drive; indigestion; inflammation of the mouth; itching; lack of muscle control; loss of appetite; loss of coordination; nausea; nervousness; numbness; perspiration; poor bladder control; rapid heartbeat; rash; reddish or brownish spots on the skin; seizures; sensitivity to light; severe muscle stiffness; sore throat; swelling of the testicles; taste disturbances; tingling sensation; tremors; vomiting; weakness; weight gain; worsening of asthma; and yellow eyes and skin.

If you experience any of these side effects or reactions, notify your doctor as soon as possible.

Important Precautions

Do not take doxepin if you are taking another type of antidepressant called a monoamine oxidase inhibitor (MAOI) or have taken one within the past two weeks, if you have a history of glaucoma or urinary retention, or if you have ever had an allergic reaction or hypersensitivity to doxepin or a similar drug.

Doxepin may make you feel dizzy and drowsy. Do not drive, operate machinery, or participate in any high-risk activities until you know exactly how the drug affects you.

Be sure to inform your doctor or dentist that you are taking doxepin before undergoing any type of surgery or dental treatment.

Food and Drug Interactions

If doxepin is taken with certain other drugs, the effects of either drug could be increased, decreased, or changed. Before beginning treatment with doxepin, tell your doctor if you are taking any other prescription or over-the-counter medications.

Combining doxepin with a MAOI can lead to extremely high fever, severe convulsions, even death. If you have been taking a MAOI, you must wait at least two weeks after discontinuing therapy with the drug before starting therapy with doxepin.

It is also important to check with your doctor before combining doxepin with cimetidine (Tagamet) and tolazamide (Tolinase).

Doxepin should not be taken with alcohol.

Recommended Dosage

Usual dosage for adults: 75 to 150 mg a day taken in one dose or several divided doses for mild to moderate depression; up to 300 mg a day for severe depression.

For elderly people, a once-a-day dosage should be determined by a doctor based on the severity of the illness.

The safety and effectiveness of doxepin use in children under the age of twelve has not been established.

Overdosage

Symptoms of an overdose of doxepin may include blurred vision; coma; convulsions; decreased intestinal movement; dilated pupils; drowsiness; excessive dryness of the mouth; high or low blood pressure; high or low body temperature; irregular or rapid heartbeat; overactive reflexes; severe breathing problems; stupor; and urinary problems. If you experience any of these symptoms, go to the nearest hospital emergency room immediately.

Pregnancy and Lactation

The safety of doxepin use during pregnancy has not been established. If you are pregnant or plan to become pregnant, notify your doctor immediately.

The drug passes into breast milk and may be harmful to a nursing infant. If the medication is essential to your health, your doctor may advise you not to breast-feed while you are taking it.

Estazolam

Brand Name
ProSom

General Information

Estazolam is a sleeping pill prescribed for the short-term treatment of insomnia. It is a member of the class of drugs called benzodiazepines, which facilitate the action of the neurotransmitter GABA (gamma-aminobutyric acid). This leads to the relaxation of the large skeletal muscles as well as a direct effect on the brain.

Insomnia may involve difficulty falling asleep, waking up frequently during the night, and waking up early and not being able to get back to sleep.

Side Effects

More common side effects may include daytime sleepiness, dizziness, lack of coordination, and sluggishness.

Less common side effects may include abdominal pain; abnormal thinking; acne; allergic reactions; back pain; body pain; changes in appetite; chest pain; chills; coldlike symptoms; confusion; cough; depression; dream abnormalities; drowsiness; dry mouth; dry skin; ear pain; excitement; eye pain; fever; gas; hangover; headache; hostility; indigestion; itching; joint pain; memory loss; muscle pain; muscle stiffness; nausea; nervousness; penile discharge; pounding heartbeat; rash; runny nose; shortness of breath; sore throat; tingling sensation; unexpected behavior changes; urinary problems; vaginal itching; vague feeling of being sick; vomiting; weakness; and weight changes.

If you experience any of these side effects or reactions, notify your doctor as soon as possible.

Important Precautions

Do not take estazolam if you have ever had an allergic reaction or hypersensitivity to it or a similar drug.

Use this medication with caution if you are older or physically run-down, if you have kidney or liver damage, or if you have breathing difficulties.

The dose of estazolam that you take at night may make you drowsy and impair your coordination the next day. Do not drive, operate machinery, or participate in any high-risk activities until you know exactly how the drug affects you.

Do not abruptly discontinue estazolam if you have ever had seizures. When ending treatment with this medication, follow your doctor's schedule for a gradual tapering of the dosage.

Estazolam is potentially addictive even when used for a relatively short time. Consequently, you may experience withdrawal symptoms when you stop taking it, including mild, temporary insomnia or irritability. Sometimes, however, more serious withdrawal symptoms such as abdominal and muscle cramps, convulsions, sweating, tremors, and vomiting occur. To help prevent withdrawal symptoms, do not abruptly discontinue estazolam. Instead, follow your doctor's schedule for a gradual tapering of the dosage.

Food and Drug Interactions

If estazolam is taken with certain other drugs, the effects of either drug could be increased, decreased, or changed. Before beginning treatment with estazolam, tell your doctor if you are taking any other prescription or over-the-counter medications.

Do not drink alcohol while taking estazolam. This combination could result in dangerously slowed breathing or coma.

For the same reason, it is important to avoid combining estazolam with any other medications that might slow the functioning of the central nervous system, including anticonvulsants, antihistamines, antipsychotics, barbiturates, monoamine oxidase inhibitors, narcotics, or sedatives.

Smokers process and eliminate estazolam relatively rapidly compared to nonsmokers.

Recommended Dosage

Usual dosage for adults: 1 mg at bedtime. Some people may need 2 mg.

Usual dosage for the elderly: 1 mg at bedtime. Some people may only require 0.5 mg.

The safety and effectiveness of estazolam in children under the age of eighteen has not been established.

Overdosage

Symptoms of an estazolam overdose may include coma, confusion, depressed breathing, drowsiness, lack of coordination, and slurred speech. If you experience any of these symptoms, go to the nearest hospital emergency room immediately.

Pregnancy and Lactation

Estazolam may cause birth defects and/or drug withdrawal symptoms in infants. As a result, it should not be taken during pregnancy. If you are pregnant or plan to become pregnant, notify your doctor immediately.

The drug is believed to pass into breast milk and may be harmful to a nursing infant. As a result, it should not be taken while breast-feeding.

Fluoxetine

Brand Name
Prozac

General Information
Fluoxetine is approved by the Food and Drug Administration for use in the treatment of depression and obsessive-compulsive disorder. It is also prescribed for the treatment of a wide variety of other conditions including attention deficit disorder, bulimia, panic disorder, borderline personality disorder, phobias, substance abuse, premenstrual syndrome, obesity, kleptomania, and addictive gambling. However, it has not been approved by the FDA for these purposes.

It is the "mother" of the class of drugs called selective serotonin reuptake inhibitors, which work by blocking the presynaptic reuptake of the neurotransmitter serotonin. This suggests that many of the symptoms of depression may result from abnormal serotonin activity in the brain.

Symptoms of depression include low, anxious, or "empty" feelings; loss of interest and pleasure in activities previously enjoyed; noticeable change of appetite; noticeable change in sleeping patterns; fatigue or loss of energy; feelings of hopelessness or pessimism; feelings of guilt, worthlessness, or helplessness; inability to concentrate, make decisions, or remember details; recurring thoughts of death or suicide, wishing to die or attempting suicide; and aches and pains, constipation, or other physical ailments that cannot be explained.

Side Effects

More common side effects may include abnormal dreams; agitation; anxiety; bronchitis; chills; diarrhea; dizziness; drowsiness; fatigue; hay fever; increased appetite; insomnia; lack or loss of appetite; light-headedness; nausea; nervousness; perspiration; tremors; weakness; weight loss; and yawning.

Less common side effects may include abnormal cessation of menstrual flow; abnormal ejaculation; abnormal gait; acne; amnesia; apathy; arthritis; asthma; belching; bone pain; breast cysts; breast pain; brief loss of consciousness; bursitis; chills; conjunctivitis; convulsions; dark, tarry stool; difficulty swallowing; dilated pupils; dimness of vision; dry skin; ear pain; eye pain; exaggerated feeling of well-being; facial swelling; fever; fluid retention; hair loss; hallucinations; hangover effect; hiccups; high or low blood pressure; hives; hostility; impotence; increased sex drive; inflammation of the esophagus, gums, mouth, stomach lining, tongue or vagina; involuntary movement; irrational ideas; irregular heartbeat; jaw or neck pain; lack of muscle coordination; low blood sugar; migraine headache; neck pain and rigidity; nosebleed; ovarian disorders; paranoid reaction; pelvic pain; pneumonia; rapid breathing; rapid heartbeat; rash; ringing in the ears; sensitivity to light; severe chest pain; skin inflammation; thirst; twitching; uncoordinated movements; urinary disorders; vague feeling of bodily discomfort; vertigo; and weight gain.

Rare side effects may include antisocial behavior; blood in urine; bloody diarrhea; bone disease; breast enlargement; cataracts; colitis; coma; deafness; decreased reflexes; dehydration; double vision; drooping of eyelids; duodenal ulcer; enlarged abdomen; enlargement of the liver; enlargement or increased activity of the thyroid gland; excess growth of coarse hair on the face and chest; excess uterine or vaginal hemorrhage; extreme muscle tension; eye bleeding; female milk production; fluid accumulation and swelling in the head; fluid buildup in the larynx and lungs; gallstones; glaucoma; gout; heart attack; hepatitis; high blood sugar; hysteria; inability to control bowel movements; increased salivation; inflammation of the eyes and eyelids, fallopian tubes, gall bladder, lungs, small intestine, testes, or tissue below the skin; kidney disorders; loss of taste; menstrual disorders; miscarriage; mouth sores; muscle inflammation or bleeding; muscle spasms; painful sexual intercourse for women; psoriasis; reddish or purplish spots on the skin; reduction of body temperature; rheumatoid arthritis; seborrhea; shingles; skin discoloration; skin inflammation and disorders; slowing of heart rate; slurred speech; spitting blood; stomach ulcer; stupor; suicidal thoughts; temporary cessation of breathing; tingling sensation around the mouth; tongue discoloration and swelling; urinary tract disorders; vomiting blood; and yellowed skin and whites of the eyes.

If you experience any of these side effects or reactions, notify your doctor as soon as possible.

Important Precautions

Serious, sometimes fatal, reactions have resulted from taking fluoxetine with another type of antidepressant called a monoamine oxidase inhibitor (MAOI) and when fluoxetine therapy is discontinued and MAOI therapy is started. Never take fluoxetine with one of these drugs or within two weeks of ending treatment with one of these drugs.

Do not take fluoxetine if you have ever had an allergic reaction or hypersensitivity to it or a similar drug.

Use this medication with caution if you have had a heart attack recently or if you have a history of kidney or liver disease, seizures, or diabetes.

Fluoxetine may make you feel dizzy and drowsy. Do not drive, operate machinery, or participate in any high-risk activities until you know exactly how the drug affects you. It might also make you feel dizzy or light-headed when getting up from a seated or prone position. If getting up slowly doesn't solve this problem, notify your doctor.

If you develop a skin rash or hives while on fluoxetine, stop taking it and inform your doctor immediately.

Food and Drug Interactions

If fluoxetine is taken with certain other drugs, the effects of either drug could be increased, decreased, or changed. Before beginning treatment with fluoxetine, tell your doctor if you are taking any other prescription or over-the-counter medications.

Fluoxetine should not be combined with MAOIs. It is also important to check with your doctor before combining fluoxetine with diazepam (Valium), digoxin (Lanoxin), drugs that act on the central nervous system, lithium (Eskalith, Lithobid), other antidepressants, the amino acid tryptophan, and warfarin (Coumadin).

Do not drink alcohol while taking fluoxetine.

Recommended Dosage

Usual dosage for adults: The usual starting dose is 20 mg a day taken in the morning. This amount may be increased after several weeks if no improvement is noticed. Dosages above 20 mg a day should be divided into two daily doses. Dosages above 80 mg a day are not recommended. It is important to note that some patients do best at less than 20 mg a day. So if a patient has not responded adequately in the 20-to-80-mg range, it is appropriate to prescribe 10 mg a day or 20 mg every other day.

Dosages for the elderly should be determined by a doctor.

The safety and effectiveness of fluoxetine use in children has not been established.

Overdosage

Symptoms of a fluoxetine overdose may include agitation, nausea, restlessness, and vomiting. If you experience any of these symptoms, go to the nearest hospital emergency room immediately.

Pregnancy and Lactation

The safety of fluoxetine use during pregnancy has not been established. If you are pregnant or plan to become pregnant, notify your doctor immediately.

Fluoxetine may pass into breast milk and may be harmful to a nursing infant. If the medication is essential to your health, your doctor may advise you not to breast-feed while you are taking it.

Fluphenazine

Brand Name

Prolixin

General Information

Fluphenazine is used in the treatment of psychotic disorders such as schizophrenia. It works by blocking the neurotransmitter dopamine. This suggests that many of the symptoms of psychosis may result from abnormal dopamine activity in the brain.

Symptoms of schizophrenia include delusions, hallucinations, disorganized speech, grossly disorganized or catatonic behavior, and absence of normal moods and emotions.

Side Effects

Fluphenazine may cause neuroleptic malignant syndrome (NMS), a rare but potentially life-threatening side effect characterized by severe muscle rigidity throughout the body. Other features of NMS include high fever, rapid heartbeat, rapid breathing, excessive perspiration, abnormal blood pressure, and kidney failure.

This drug may also cause a serious and at times permanent side effect called tardive dyskinesia. This neurological syndrome results in involuntary movements of the mouth, lips, and tongue such as tongue rolling, lip licking and smacking, chewing or sucking motions, pouting, and grimacing.

Other side effects may include abnormal muscle rigidity; abnormalities of movement and posture;

altered mental state; asthma; blood disorders; blurred vision; bowel movements that are large and hard; breast development in males; chewing movements; complete or almost complete loss of movement; constipation; dizziness; drowsiness; dry mouth; excessive or spontaneous flow of milk; excessive urine; excitement; eye problems; eyeball rotation or state of fixed gaze; fluid accumulation in the brain; fluid retention and swelling; glaucoma; headache; heart attack; high blood pressure; high fever; hives; impotence; inability to sit still; increased sex drive in women; intestinal blockage; irregular blood pressure, pulse, and heartbeat; irregular menstrual periods; loss of appetite; masklike facial expression and rigidity; nasal congestion; nausea; oily scalp; painful muscle spasms; protruding tongue; puckering of the mouth; puffing of the cheeks; rapid heartbeat; red blood spots; restlessness; salivation; sensitivity to light; skin inflammation and peeling; skin itching, pigmentation, rash, lesions, and crusts; sluggishness; sore throat, mouth, and gums; strange dreams; sweating; swelling of the throat; twitching in the body, neck, shoulders, and face; visual problems; weight change; and yellowing of the skin and whites of the eyes.

If you experience any of these side effects or reactions, notify your doctor as soon as possible.

Important Precautions

Keep in mind that fluphenazine can cause neuroleptic malignant syndrome and tardive dyskinesia.

Do not take fluphenazine if you are also taking central nervous system depressants, if you have had brain or liver damage, or if you have a bone-marrow or blood disorder.

Use this medication with caution if you have a history of breast cancer, convulsive disorders, heart or kidney disease, seizures, or certain tumors. Fluphenazine should also be used cautiously by people who are exposed to extreme heat or pesticides.

Periodic evaluations of your blood, liver, and kidneys should be performed throughout treatment.

Fluphenazine may make you feel dizzy and drowsy. Do not drive, operate machinery, or participate in any high-risk activities until you know exactly how the drug affects you.

Abruptly discontinuing fluphenazine may result in dizziness, nausea, stomach inflammation, tremors, and vomiting. When ending treatment with this medication, follow your doctor's schedule for a gradual withdrawal.

Food and Drug Interactions

If fluphenazine is taken with certain other drugs, the effects of either drug could be increased, decreased, or changed. Before beginning treatment with fluphenazine, tell your doctor if you are taking any other prescription or over-the-counter medications.

It is particularly important to check with your doctor before taking fluphenazine with analgesics, antihistamines, atropine (Donnatal), barbiturates, or epinephrine, which is often used for the emergency treatment of severe allergic reactions.

Fluphenazine should not be combined with alcohol, narcotics, sleeping pills, or tranquilizers.

Recommended Dosage

Usual dosage for adults: The usual starting dose is 2.5 to 10 mg a day taken in three or four divided doses spaced six to eight hours apart. If necessary, this amount may be increased to 40 mg a day. Once symptoms are under control, the dosage may gradually be lowered. Maintenance doses typically range from 1 to 5 mg a day.

Usual dosage for the elderly: The usual starting dose is 1 to 2.5 mg a day since elderly people have a higher risk of developing tardive dyskinesia.

Dosages for children should be individually tailored by a doctor.

Overdosage

Symptoms of a fluphenazine overdose depend on the amount ingested and individual patient tolerance. If you suspect an overdose, go to the nearest hospital emergency room immediately.

Pregnancy and Lactation

Fluphenazine should only be used during pregnancy if the potential benefits clearly outweigh any potential risks to the fetus. If you are pregnant or plan to become pregnant, notify your doctor immediately.

The drug may pass into breast milk and may be harmful to a nursing infant. If the medication is essential to your health, your doctor may advise you not to breast-feed while you are taking it.

Flurazepam

Brand Name
Dalmane

General Information
Flurazepam is a sleeping pill prescribed for the short-term treatment of insomnia. It is a member of the class of drugs called benzodiazepines, which facilitate the action of the neurotransmitter GABA (gamma-aminobutyric acid). This leads to the relaxation of the large skeletal muscles as well as a direct effect on the brain.

Insomnia may involve difficulty falling asleep, waking up frequently during the night, and waking up early and not being able to get back to sleep.

Side Effects
More common side effects may include dizziness, drowsiness, falling, lack of coordination, light-headedness, and staggering.

Less common or rare side effects may include abdominal pain; apprehension; bitter taste; blood disorder; blurred vision; body and joint pain; burning eyes; chest pains; confusion; constipation; depression; diarrhea; difficulty in focusing; dry mouth; exaggerated feeling of well-being; excessive salivation; excitement; faintness; flushes; genital and urinary tract disorders; hallucinations; headache; heartburn; hyperactivity; irritability; itching; loss of appetite; low blood pressure; nausea; nervousness; palpitations; rash; restlessness; shortness of breath; slurred speech; stimulation;

stomach upset; sweating; talkativeness; vomiting; and weakness.

If you experience any of these side effects or reactions, notify your doctor as soon as possible.

Important Precautions

Do not take flurazepam if you have ever had an allergic reaction or hypersensitivity to it or a similar drug.

Use this medication with caution if you are severely depressed or have a history of severe depression, if you have decreased kidney or liver function, or if you have chronic respiratory disease. If you suffer from any of these conditions, be sure to discuss the details thoroughly with your doctor before taking flurazepam.

Flurazepam may make you drowsy or less alert. Do not drive, operate machinery, or participate in any high-risk activities until you know exactly how the drug affects you.

This medication is potentially addictive even when used for a relatively short time. Consequently, you may experience withdrawal symptoms when you stop taking it. Withdrawal symptoms may include abdominal and muscle cramps, convulsions, depressed mood, insomnia, sweating, tremors, and vomiting. To help prevent withdrawal symptoms, do not abruptly discontinue flurazepam. Instead, follow your doctor's schedule for a gradual tapering of the dosage.

Food and Drug Interactions

If flurazepam is taken with certain other drugs, the effects of either drug could be increased, decreased, or changed. Before beginning treatment with flurazepam, tell your doctor if you are taking any other prescription or over-the-counter medications.

It is particularly important to avoid combining flurazepam with antihistamines or any other medications that might slow the functioning of the central nervous system.

Do not drink alcohol while taking flurazepam.

Recommended Dosage

Usual dosage for adults: 30 mg at bedtime. Some people may only require 15 mg. The dosage should be tailored to the individual.

Usual dosage for the elderly: The dosage should be limited to the minimum effective amount. The usual starting dose is 15 mg at bedtime.

The safety and effectiveness of flurazepam in children under the age of fifteen has not been established.

Overdosage

Symptoms of a flurazepam overdose may include coma, confusion, low blood pressure, and sleepiness. If you experience any of these symptoms, go to the nearest hospital emergency room immediately.

Pregnancy and Lactation

Flurazepam may cause birth defects. As a result, it should not be taken during pregnancy. If you are pregnant or plan to become pregnant, notify your doctor immediately.

The drug may pass into breast milk and may be harmful to a nursing infant. If the medication is essential to your health, your doctor may advise you not to breast-feed while you are taking it.

Fluvoxamine

Brand Name

Luvox

General Information

Fluvoxamine is used in the treatment of obsessive-compulsive disorder. It is a member of the class of drugs called selective serotonin reuptake inhibitors, which work by blocking the presynaptic reuptake of the neurotransmitter serotonin. This suggests that many of the symptoms of obsessive-compulsive disorder may result from abnormal serotonin activity in the brain.

Obsessions are intrusive, unwanted ideas, images, impulses, or worries that dominate a person's thoughts, such as avoiding contamination or doubting whether the front door is locked. Compulsions are senseless, irrational rituals that a person feels driven to perform again and again, such as washing hands or checking the front door dozens of times a day.

Side Effects

More common side effects may include abdominal pain; abnormal ejaculation; accidental injury; agitation; amnesia; anorexia; anxiety; apathy; decreased libido; decreased muscular movement; diarrhea; dizziness; dry mouth; elevated liver enzymes; headache; hypertension; inability to achieve orgasm; increased cough; increased muscular movement; insomnia; lack or loss of strength; low blood pressure; malaise; mania; muscle twitching or spasms; nausea; nervousness; painful digestion; psychotic reaction; rapid heartbeat; rhinitis; sinus inflammation; sleepiness; strange taste in mouth; sweating; swelling; temporary loss of consciousness; tremors; urinary frequency; vomiting; and weight gain or loss.

Less common side effects may include abnormal decrease in the number of blood platelets; abnormal involuntary movements; abnormal vision; acne; agoraphobia; alteration of the sense of smell; anemia; arthritis; asthma; belching; black feces; bleeding from the stomach or intestinal tract; bleeding from the uterus; blood in the urine; boils; breast pain; bronchitis; bursitis; cardiovascular disease; central nervous system depression; chest pain; cold extremities; conjunctivitis; convulsions; deafness; defective muscular coordination; dehydration; delayed menstruation; delirium; delusions; depersonalization; disease of the lymph nodes; double vision; drug dependence; dry eyes; dry skin; ear pain; eczema; emotional changes; euphoria; excessive menstrual bleeding; excessive sleeping; excessive urination; excessive urination during the night; eye pain; hallucinations; hair loss; heart failure; hemorrhoids; high cholesterol; hoarseness; hostility; hyperventilation; hypochondria; hypothyroidism; hysteria; imparied urination; inability to sit still; incoordination; increase in the number of white blood cells; increased salivation; increased sex drive; inflammation of a tendon sheath; inflammation of the bladder, colon, esophagus, gums, intestinal tract, middle ear, mouth, stomach, tongue, or vagina; irregular pulse; joint pain; lack of urine formation; lactation; loss of taste; menopause; muscle spasms; muscular weakness and abnormal fatigue; myocardial infarction; neck pain; neck rigidity; nosebleed; painful or difficult urination; paleness; paralysis of one side of the body; paranoid reaction; premenstrual syndrome; prolonged muscle contractions; pronounced or abnormal dilation of the pupils; psychosis; rectal hemorrhage; red and scaly skin; seborrhea; sensitivity to light; severe pain along the course of a nerve; skin discoloration; sleep disorder; slow heartbeat; stomach or intestinal ulcer; stupor; suicide attempt; twitching; unsteady gait; unusual intolerance to light; urinary incontinence; urinary tract infection; vaginal hemorrhage; vertigo; and visual field defect.

Rare side effects may include abnormal decrease of white blood cells; blood in the semen; coma; complete or partial loss of muscle movement; congestion of upper airway; contraction of the chewing muscles; corneal ulcer; coronary artery disease; coughing up blood; cysts; decreased amount of urine formation; decreased reflexes; deformity of the neck; detached retina; diabetes mellitus; embolus; enlargement of the thyroid gland; extreme potassium depletion; fecal incontinence; fibrillations; gallstones; hiccups; high or low blood sugar; inability to speak; increase of lipids in the blood; infarction in the lung; inflammation of a vein, the gallbladder, or pericardium; intestinal obstruction; jaundice; joint disease; kidney stones; obsessions; obstructive pulmonary disease; pelvic pain; pneumonia; slurred speech; spasm of the larynx; stroke; sudden death; tardive dyskinesia; temporary cessation of breathing; vomiting of blood; and withdrawal syndrome.

If you experience any of these side effects or reactions, notify your doctor as soon as possible.

Important Precautions

Serious, sometimes fatal, reactions have resulted from taking fluvoxamine with a type of antidepressant called a monoamine oxidase inhibitor (MAOI) and when fluvoxamine therapy is discontinued and MAOI therapy is started. Never take fluvoxamine with one of these drugs or within two weeks of ending treatment with one of these drugs.

Do not take fluvoxamine if you have ever had an allergic reaction or hypersensitivity to it or a similar drug.

Use this medication with caution if you have a history of liver disease, mania, or seizures.

Fluvoxamine may make you feel dizzy and drowsy. Do not drive, operate machinery, or participate in any high-risk activities until you know exactly how the drug affects you.

Notify your doctor if you develop a rash, hives, or a related allergic reaction during treatment.

Food and Drug Interactions

If fluvoxamine is taken with certain other drugs, the effects of either drug could be increased, decreased, or changed. Before beginning treatment with fluvoxamine, tell your doctor if you are taking any other prescription or over-the-counter medications.

Fluvoxamine should not be combined with MAOIs, astemizole (Hismanal), or terfenadine (Seldane). It is also important to check with your doctor before combining fluvoxamine with alprazolam (Xanax), carbamazepine (Atretol, Tegretol), clozapine (Clozaril), diltiazem (Cardizem), lithium (Eskalith, Lithobid), metoprolol (Lopressor), propranolol (Inderal), theophylline (Theo-Dur), warfarin (Coumadin), the amino acid tryptophan, or tricyclic antidepressants.

Do not drink alcohol while taking fluvoxamine.

Recommended Dosage

Usual dosage for adults: The usual starting dose is 50 mg a day taken in a single dose at bedtime. If necessary, this amount may be increased by 50-mg increments until the maximum therapeutic benefit is achieved. Dosages above 300 mg a day are not recommended.

Elderly people and individuals with liver damage are typically treated with lower doses.

The safety and effectiveness of fluvoxamine use in children under the age of eighteen has not been established.

Overdosage

An overdose of fluvoxamine can be fatal. Common symptoms of overdose include diarrhea, dizziness, drowsiness, and vomiting. Other signs include coma, convulsions, liver function abnormalities, low blood pressure, rapid heartbeat, respiratory difficulties, and slow heartbeat. If you experience any of these symptoms, go to the nearest hospital emergency room immediately.

Pregnancy and Lactation

The safety of fluvoxamine use during pregnancy has not been established. If you are pregnant or plan to become pregnant, notify your doctor immediately.

Fluvoxamine passes into breast milk and may be harmful to a nursing infant. If the medication is essential to your health, your doctor may advise you not to breast-feed while you are taking it.

Haloperidol

Brand Name
Haldol

General Information
Haloperidol is used in the treatment of psychotic disorders such as schizophrenia. It works by blocking the neurotransmitter dopamine. This suggests that many of the symptoms of psychosis may result from abnormal dopamine activity in the brain.

Symptoms of schizophrenia include delusions, hallucinations, disorganized speech, grossly disorganized or catatonic behavior, and absence of normal moods and emotions.

Side Effects
Haloperidol may cause neuroleptic malignant syndrome (NMS), a rare but potentially life-threatening side effect characterized by severe muscle rigidity throughout the body. Other features of NMS include high fever, rapid heartbeat, rapid breathing, excessive

perspiration, abnormal blood pressure, and kidney failure.

This drug may also cause a serious and at times permanent side effect called tardive dyskinesia. This neurological syndrome results in involuntary movements of the mouth, lips, and tongue such as tongue rolling, lip licking and smacking, chewing or sucking motions, pouting, and grimacing.

Other side effects may include abnormal secretion of milk; agitation; anemia; anxiety; appetite changes; blurred vision; breast development in males; breast pain; cataracts; catatonic state; chewing movements; confusion; constipation; coughing; deeper breathing; dehydration; depression; diarrhea; dizziness; drowsiness; dry mouth; exaggerated feeling of well-being; exaggerated reflexes; excessive salivation; fever; hair loss; hallucinations; headache; heat stroke; high or low blood sugar; impotence; increased sex drive; indigestion; involuntary movements; irregular blood pressure, pulse, and heartbeat; irregular menstrual periods; lack of muscular coordination; muscle spasms; nausea; Parkinson-like symptoms; persistent, abnormal erections; physical rigidity and stupor; protruding tongue; puckering of the mouth; puffing of the cheeks; rapid heartbeat; restlessness; rigid arms, feet, head, and muscles; rotation of the eyeballs; seizures; sensitivity to light; skin rash and eruptions; sleeplessness; sluggishness; sweating; swelling of breasts; twitching in the body, neck, shoulders, and face; urinary retention; vertigo; visual problems; vomiting; wheezing or asthmalike symptoms; and yellowing of the skin and whites of the eyes.

If you experience any of these side effects or reactions, notify your doctor as soon as possible.

Important Precautions

Keep in mind that haloperidol can cause neuroleptic malignant syndrome and tardive dyskinesia.

Do not take haloperidol if you have Parkinson's disease, if you are also taking central nervous system depressants, or if you are hypersensitive to haloperidol.

Use this medication with caution if you have a history of breast cancer, cardiovascular disease, chest pain, glaucoma, seizures, or an allergy to this type of drug.

Haloperidol may make you feel dizzy and drowsy. Do not drive, operate machinery, or participate in any high-risk activities until you know exactly how the drug affects you.

Abruptly discontinuing haloperidol may result in temporary muscle spasms and twitches. When ending treatment with this medication, follow your doctor's schedule for a gradual withdrawal.

Food and Drug Interactions

If haloperidol is taken with certain other drugs, the effects of either drug could be increased, decreased, or changed. Before beginning treatment with haloperidol, tell your doctor if you are taking any other prescription or over-the-counter medications.

It is particularly important to check with your doctor before taking haloperidol with anticoagulants, anticonvulsants, epinephrine (which is often used in the emergency treatment of severe allergic reactions), or lithium (Eskalith, Lithobid).

Haloperidol should not be combined with alcohol, narcotics, sleeping pills, or tranquilizers.

Recommended Dosage

Usual dosage for adults: 1 to 6 mg a day taken in two or three divided doses for moderate symptoms; 6 to 15 mg a day taken in two or three divided doses for severe symptoms.

Elderly people usually take lower doses of haloperidol since they have a higher risk of developing tardive dyskinesia.

Usual dosage for children aged three to twelve: .05 to .15 mg per kilogram of body weight per day. Haloperidol is not recommended for children under the age of three.

Overdosage

Symptoms of a haloperidol overdose may include catatonic state, coma, decreased breathing, low blood pressure, rigid muscles, sedation, tremors, and weakness. If you experience any of these symptoms, go to the nearest hospital emergency room immediately.

Pregnancy and Lactation

The safety of haloperidol use during pregnancy has not been established. As a result, it should only be taken during pregnancy if the potential benefits clearly outweigh any potential risks to the fetus. If you are pregnant or plan to become pregnant, notify your doctor immediately.

The drug should not be used while breast-feeding.

Imipramine

Brand Name
Tofranil

General Information

Imipramine is used in the treatment of depression and panic disorder. It is a member of the class of drugs called tricyclic antidepressants, which work by blocking the presynaptic reuptake of the neurotransmitters serotonin, norepinephrine, and dopamine in the brain. This suggests that many of the symptoms of depression may result from imbalances of one or more of these neurotransmitters.

Symptoms of depression include low, anxious, or "empty" feelings; loss of interest and pleasure in activities previously enjoyed; noticeable change of appetite; noticeable change in sleeping patterns; fatigue or loss of energy; feelings of hopelessness or pessimism; feelings of guilt, worthlessness, or helplessness; inability to concentrate, make decisions, or remember details; recurring thoughts of death or suicide, wishing to die or attempting suicide; and aches and pains, constipation, or other physical ailments that cannot be explained.

Side Effects

Side effects may include abdominal cramps; agitation; anxiety; black tongue; bleeding sores; blood disorders; blurred vision; breast development in males; confusion; constipation or diarrhea; cough;

delusions; dilated pupils; disorientation; dizziness; drowsiness; dry mouth; episodes of elation or irritability; excessive or spontaneous flow of milk, fatigue; fever; flushing; frequent urination or difficulty or delay in urinating; hair loss; hallucinations; headache; heart attack; heart failure; high blood pressure; high or low blood sugar; hives; impotence; increased or decreased sex drive; increased pressure in the eyes; inflammation of the mouth; insomnia; intestinal blockage; lack of coordination; light-headedness; loss of appetite; nausea; nightmares; numbness in the hands and feet; odd taste in mouth; pounding heart; purplish or reddish brown spots on the skin; rapid heartbeat; restlessness; ringing in the ears; seizures; sensitivity to light; skin itching and rash; sore throat; stomach pain; stroke; sweating; swelling in the face or tongue; swelling of the breasts or testicles; swollen glands; tendency to fall; tingling; tremors; visual problems; vomiting; weakness; weight gain or loss; and yellowed skin and whites of eyes.

If you experience any of these side effects or reactions, notify your doctor as soon as possible.

Important Precautions

Do not take imipramine if you have had a heart attack recently, if you are taking a type of antidepressant called a monoamine oxidase inhibitor (MAOI), or if you have ever had an allergic reaction or hypersensitivity to imipramine or a similar drug.

Use this medication with caution if you have a history of heart, liver, kidney, or thyroid disease, narrow-angle glaucoma or increased pressure in the eyes, seizures, or urinary retention.

Imipramine may make you feel dizzy and drowsy.

Do not drive, operate machinery, or participate in any high-risk activities until you know exactly how the drug affects you.

If you develop a sore throat or fever while taking imipramine, be sure to inform your doctor.

Since imipramine can make you sensitive to light, try to stay out of the sun as much as possible during your treatment.

Abruptly discontinuing imipramine may result in headaches, nausea, and malaise. When ending treatment with this medication, follow your doctor's schedule for a gradual withdrawal.

Food and Drug Interactions

If imipramine is taken with certain other drugs, the effects of either drug could be increased, decreased, or changed. Before beginning treatment with imipramine, tell your doctor if you are taking any other prescription or over-the-counter medications.

Imipramine should not be combined with MAOIs. It is also important to check with your doctor before taking imipramine with anticholinergic drugs such as Artane and Cogentin, antihypertensive drugs, decongestants, thyroid medications, albuterol (Proventil, Ventolin), carbamazepine (Tegretol), cimetidine (Tagamet), clonidine (Catapres), desipramine (Norpramin), epinephrine (Epipen), fluoxetine (Prozac), guanethidine (Ismelin), or methylphenidate (Ritalin).

Imipramine should not be taken with alcohol, sleeping pills, tranquilizers, or narcotic painkillers.

Recommended Dosage

Usual dosage for adults: 50 to 150 mg a day with a total daily limit of 200 mg.

Usual dosage for adolescents and the elderly: 40 to 100 mg a day.

Dosages for children should be individually tailored by a physician.

Overdosage

An overdose of imipramine can be fatal. Symptoms of overdose may include agitation; bluish skin; coma; convulsions; difficulty breathing; dilated pupils; drowsiness; heart failure; high fever; involuntary writhing or jerking movements; irregular or rapid heartbeat; lack of coordination; overactive reflexes; restlessness; rigid muscles, shock, stupor, sweating, and vomiting. If you experience any of these symptoms, go to the nearest hospital emergency room immediately.

Pregnancy and Lactation

Imipramine should only be used during pregnancy if the potential benefits clearly outweigh any potential risks to the fetus. If you are pregnant or plan to become pregnant, notify your doctor immediately.

The drug may pass into breast milk and may be harmful to a nursing infant. If the medication is essential to your health, your doctor may advise you not to breast-feed while you are taking it.

Lithium

Brand Names

Cibalith-S, Eskalith, Eskalith-CR, Lithane, Lithobid, Lithonate, Lithotabs

General Information

Lithium is prescribed in the treatment of bipolar or manic-depressive illness. It is used to treat the manic phase of the disorder as well as to prevent the recurrence of both manic and depressive episodes in stabilized patients. No one knows exactly how lithium works. Scientists believe that chemical imbalances in certain brain cells responsible for emotions and behavior are at the root of manic-depressive illness and that lithium corrects those imbalances.

Symptoms of mania include elation, hyperactivity, flight of ideas, rapid speech, grandiose ideas, hostility, decreased need for sleep, and uncharacteristically poor judgment. Once the mania subsides, lithium is administered on a maintenance basis, at a somewhat lower dosage, to reduce the frequency and severity of future manic episodes. Lithium prevents the recurrence of depressive episodes as well. However, antidepressants are frequently required to treat "breakthrough" depressions.

Side Effects

Common side effects may include diarrhea; drowsiness; fatigue; fever; frequent urination; headache; increased thirst; minor memory impairments; muscle weakness; slight hand tremor; vomiting; and weight gain.

Less common side effects may include abnormal heartbeat; blackout spells; blurred vision; collapsed blood vessels; coma; confusion; dehydration; dizziness; dry hair; dry mouth; dry skin; excessive thirst; goiter; hair follicle infections; hair loss; incontinence; involuntary eyeball movement; itching; lack of coordination; lack of sensation in the skin; lethargy; loss of appetite; low blood pressure; metallic taste; muscle irritability; nausea; physical and mental slowness; restlessness; seizures; skin ulcers; sleepiness; slurred speech; stupor; swelling of the ankles or wrists; temporary blind spot in the eye; underactive or overactive thyroid; unusual weight gain or loss; vertigo; and writhing movements.

If you experience any of these side effects or reactions, notify your doctor as soon as possible.

Important Precautions

If the dosage of lithium is too low, you will not derive any benefit. If the dosage is too high, you will experience unwanted side effects. In order to determine a dosage that is both safe and effective, your doctor will check the level of lithium in your blood at least once a week when the drug is first prescribed. Once the blood levels have stabilized, the test will be repeated on a regular basis for as long as you are taking the medication.

Since there is a thin line between the dosage of lithium that works well and the dosage that produces overdose effects, it is important to monitor yourself for adverse reactions and report any new symptoms to your doctor immediately.

During the first few days of treatment, lithium may make you feel dizzy and drowsy. Do not drive a car, operate dangerous machinery, or perform hazardous tasks until you know exactly how the drug affects you.

Use lithium with extreme caution if you have kidney disease, cardiovascular disease, severe dehydration, or sodium depletion. To prevent dehydration, drink ten to twelve glasses of water or fluids a day and maintain your salt intake. If prolonged sweating or diarrhea occurs, your doctor may recommend extra fluids and salt. If you develop an infection that causes fever, diarrhea, or vomiting, he may advise you to reduce your lithium dosage or stop taking it temporarily.

Be sure to have your kidney function monitored routinely.

Food and Drug Interactions

If lithium is taken with certain other drugs, the effects of either drug could be increased, decreased, or changed. Before beginning treatment with lithium, tell your doctor if you are taking any other prescription or over-the-counter medications.

It is particularly important to check with your doctor before combining lithium with antipsychotic drugs, ACE-inhibitor blood-pressure drugs such as Capoten and Vasotec, anti-inflammatory drugs, asthma drugs, bicarbonate of soda, diuretics, or iodine-containing preparations such as Pima syrup.

Lithium may also prolong or intensify the effects of certain drugs used in anesthesia. If you are undergoing an operation, make sure the surgeon and anesthesiologist know you are taking the medication.

Recommended Dosage

The recommended adult daily dose of lithium depends upon whether it is being used to treat manic episodes or for maintenance. The dosage must also be individualized based on the serum lithium level, which is determined with a blood test. As a result, a doctor may prescribe more or less than the following rough guidelines.

Usual adult dosage for manic episodes: 900 mg twice a day or 600 mg three times a day for a total of 1,800 mg a day.

Usual adult dosage for maintenance: 900 to 1,200 mg a day in two or three divided doses.

Elderly people usually respond to lower dosages of lithium and may show signs of overdose at blood levels normally tolerated by younger people.

Lithium is not recommended for children under the age of twelve.

Overdosage

Initial signs of lithium overdose include loss of appetite, vomiting, diarrhea, blurred vision, drowsiness, sluggishness, giddiness, trembling, lack of coordination, and slurred speech. A more severe overdose may result in fainting, seizures, stiffened limbs, psychotic thinking, psychosis, coma, or even death. If you experience any of these symptoms, go to the nearest hospital emergency room immediately.

Pregnancy and Lactation

Using lithium during pregnancy is generally not recommended due to the slight possibility that it might cause birth defects. If you are pregnant or plan to become pregnant, notify your doctor immediately.

Lithium passes into breast milk and may be harmful to a nursing infant. In particular, it may cause dehydration. If the drug is essential to your health, your doctor may advise you not to breast-feed while you are taking it.

Lorazepam

Brand Name

Ativan

General Information

Lorazepam is used in the treatment of anxiety disorder and panic disorder. It is a member of the class of drugs called benzodiazepines, which facilitate the action of the neurotransmitter GABA (gamma-aminobutyric acid). Benzodiazepines decrease anxiety via direct effects on the brain. They may also make you drowsy depending upon which one you take and how much you take. Benzodiazepines can relax skeletal muscles as well.

Symptoms of anxiety include trembling, twitching, heart palpitations, shortness of breath, sweaty palms, clammy skin, dry mouth, dizziness, nausea, and trouble swallowing.

Side Effects

More common side effects may include dizziness, unsteadiness, and weakness.

Less common or rare side effects may include agitation, change in appetite, depression, disorientation, eye function disorders, headache, impaired memory, nausea, sleep disturbances, and stomach and intestinal disorders.

If you experience any of these side effects or reactions, notify your doctor as soon as possible.

Important Precautions

Do not take lorazepam if you have narrow-angle glaucoma or if you have ever had an allergic reaction or hypersensitivity to lorazepam or a similar drug.

Use this medication with caution if you are severely depressed or have a history of severe depression, or if you suffer from decreased kidney or liver function.

Lorazepam may make you drowsy or less alert. Do not drive, operate machinery, or participate in any high-risk activities until you know exactly how the drug affects you.

Abruptly discontinuing lorazepam may result in withdrawal symptoms such as abdominal and muscle cramps, convulsions, depressed mood, insomnia, perspiration, tremors, and vomiting. When ending treatment with this medication, follow your doctor's schedule for a gradual withdrawal.

Food and Drug Interactions

If lorazepam is taken with certain other drugs, the effects of either drug could be increased, decreased, or changed. Before beginning treatment with lorazepam, tell your doctor if you are taking any other prescription or over-the-counter medications.

It is particularly important to check with your doctor before combining lorazepam with barbiturates or other sedatives.

Do not drink alcohol while taking lorazepam.

Recommended Dosage

Usual dosage for adults: The usual starting dosage is 2 to 3 mg a day taken in two or three doses. If necessary, this amount may be gradually increased until an effective dose is reached. The average dose is 2 to 6 mg a day.

Usual dosage for the elderly: The usual starting dosage is 1 to 2 mg a day taken in several divided doses. This dosage may be adjusted by a doctor as needed.

The safety and effectiveness of lorazepam in children under the age of twelve has not been established.

Overdosage

Symptoms of a lorazepam overdose may include coma, confusion, low blood pressure, and sleepiness. If you experience any of these symptoms, go to the nearest hospital emergency room immediately.

Pregnancy and Lactation

Lorazepam may cause birth defects. As a result, it should not be taken during pregnancy. If you are pregnant or plan to become pregnant, notify your doctor immediately.

The drug may pass into breast milk and may be harmful to a nursing infant. If the medication is essential to your health, your doctor may advise you not to breast-feed while you are taking it.

Loxapine

Brand Name

Loxitane

General Information

Loxapine is used in the treatment of psychotic disorders such as schizophrenia. It works by blocking the neurotransmitter dopamine. This suggests that many of the symptoms of psychosis may result from abnormal dopamine activity in the brain.

Symptoms of schizophrenia include delusions, hallucinations, disorganized speech, grossly disorganized or catatonic behavior, and absence of normal moods and emotions.

Side Effects

Loxapine may cause neuroleptic malignant syndrome (NMS), a rare but potentially life-threatening side effect characterized by severe muscle rigidity throughout the body. Other features of NMS include high fever, rapid heartbeat, rapid breathing, excessive perspiration, abnormal blood pressure, and kidney failure.

This drug may also cause a serious and at times permanent side effect called tardive dyskinesia. This neurological syndrome results in involuntary movements of the mouth, lips, and tongue such as tongue rolling, lip licking and smacking, chewing or sucking motions, pouting, and grimacing.

Other side effects may include agitation; blood disorders; blurred vision; complete or partial loss of muscle movement; confusion; constipation; dandruff; dermatitis; difficulty in breathing; dizziness; drowsiness; dry mouth; excessive salivation; excessive thirst; fainting; flushing; hair loss; headache; high blood pressure; high fever; insomnia; involuntary fixation of the eyeballs; light-headedness; low blood pressure; masklike facial expression; muscle twitching; nasal congestion; nausea; numbness; paralysis of the intestines; puffiness of the face; rapid heartbeat; rash; rigidity; seizures; sensation of internal restlessness; sensation of numbness or tingling; severe and painful spasms of muscles in the head and neck; severe itching; shuffling gait; slurred speech; staggering gait; temporary loss of consciousness; tension; tongue protrusion; tremors; urinary retention; vomiting; weakness; and weight gain or loss.

If you experience any of these side effects or reactions, notify your doctor as soon as possible.

Important Precautions

Keep in mind that loxapine can cause neuroleptic malignant syndrome and tardive dyskinesia.

Do not take loxapine if you have ever had an allergic reaction or hypersensitivity to it or a similar drug.

Use this medication with caution if you have a history of breast cancer, cardiovascular disease, glaucoma, seizures, or urinary retention.

Loxapine may inhibit the vomiting reflex. As a result, it may mask the symptoms of drug overdose, brain tumors, intestinal blockage, and other conditions.

This drug may make you feel drowsy and impair your coordination. Do not drive, operate machinery, or participate in any high-risk activities until you know exactly how it affects you.

Food and Drug Interactions

If loxapine is taken with certain other drugs, the effects of either drug could be increased, decreased, or changed. Before beginning treatment with loxapine, tell your doctor if you are taking any other prescription or over-the-counter medications.

Loxapine should not be combined with alcohol, narcotics, sleeping pills, or tranquilizers.

Recommended Dosage

Usual dosage for adults: The usual starting dose is 10 mg two times a day. Severely disturbed individuals, however, may need to take up to 50 mg a day. Dosages should then be increased fairly rapidly over a seven- to ten-day period until psychotic symptoms are under control. The usual daily maintenance dose typically ranges from 60 to 100 mg. Dosages above 250 mg a day are not recommended.

The safety and effectiveness of loxapine use in children under the age of sixteen has not been established.

Overdosage

Symptoms of a loxapine overdose depend on the amount ingested and individual patient tolerance. They may range from mild depression of the central nervous system and cardiovascular system to severe hypertension, respiratory depression, unconsciousness, convulsive seizures, and kidney failure. If you experience any of these symptoms, go to the nearest hospital emergency room immediately.

Pregnancy and Lactation

The safety of loxapine use during pregnancy has not been established. As a result, it should only be taken during pregnancy if the potential benefits clearly outweigh any potential risks to the fetus. If you are pregnant or plan to become pregnant, notify your doctor immediately.

Studies have also not determined the safety of using loxapine during lactation. Consequently, the drug should only be used by a nursing mother if the potential benefits of therapy clearly outweigh any potential risks to the infant.

Maprotiline

Brand Name
Ludiomil

General Information

Maprotiline is used in the treatment of depression and anxiety associated with depression. It is also used to treat the depressive phase of manic-depressive illness. Maprotiline is a tetracyclic antidepressant, which works by blocking the presynaptic reuptake of the neurotransmitters serotonin, norepinephrine, and dopamine in the brain. This suggests that many of the symptoms of depression may result from imbalances of one or more of these neurotransmitters.

Symptoms of depression include low, anxious, or "empty" feelings; loss of interest and pleasure in activities previously enjoyed; noticeable change of appetite; noticeable change in sleeping patterns; fatigue or loss of energy; feelings of hopelessness or pessimism; feelings of guilt, worthlessness, or helplessness; inability to concentrate, make decisions, or remember details; recurring thoughts of death or suicide, wishing to die or attempting suicide; and aches and pains, constipation, or other physical ailments that cannot be explained.

Side Effects

More common side effects may include agitation, anxiety, blurred vision, constipation, dizziness, drowsiness, dry mouth, fatigue, headache, insomnia, nausea, nervousness, tremors, and weakness.

Rare side effects may include abdominal cramps; allergies; bitter taste in the mouth; black tongue; bleeding sores; blocked intestine; breast development in males; breast enlargement in females; confusion; decreased memory; delusions; diarrhea; difficult or frequent urination; difficulty swallowing; dilated pupils; disorientation; excessive or spontaneous flow of milk; excessive perspiration; fainting, feeling of unreality; fever; flushing, hair loss; hallucinations; heart attack; high blood pressure; high or low blood sugar; impotence; increased or decreased sex drive; increased psychotic symptoms; increased salivation; inflammation of the mouth; involuntary movement; irregular or rapid heartbeat; mania; nasal congestion; nightmares; numbness; overactivity; palpitations; red, black, or blue spots on the skin; restlessness; ringing in the ears; seizures; sensitivity to light; skin itching and rash; speech difficulty; stomach pain; stroke; swelling due to fluid retention; swelling of the testicles; tingling; twitches; unstable movements and gait; vomiting; weight gain or loss; and yellowish skin tone.

If you experience any of these side effects or reactions, notify your doctor as soon as possible.

Important Precautions

Do not take maprotiline if you have had a heart attack recently, if you are taking a type of antidepressant called a monoamine oxidase inhibitor (MAOI) or have taken one within the past two weeks, if you have had seizures, or if you have ever had an allergic reaction or hypersensitivity to maprotiline or a similar drug.

Use this medication with caution if you have a

history of glaucoma, heart disease, heart attacks, thyroid disease, or difficult urination.

Studies have linked maprotiline to seizures, especially when taken in amounts larger than prescribed or when taken with antipsychotic drugs.

Maprotiline may make you feel dizzy and drowsy. Do not drive, operate machinery, or participate in any high-risk activities until you know exactly how the drug affects you.

Since this drug can make you sensitive to light, try to stay out of the sun as much as possible during your treatment.

Food and Drug Interactions

If maprotiline is taken with certain other drugs, the effects of either drug could be increased, decreased, or changed. Before beginning treatment with maprotiline, tell your doctor if you are taking any other prescription or over-the-counter medications.

Maprotiline should not be combined with MAOIs. It is also important to check with your doctor before taking maprotiline with anticholinergic drugs, antipsychotic drugs, benzodiazepines, thyroid medications, albuterol (Proventil, Ventolin), cimetidine (Tagamet), and guanethidine (Ismelin).

Maprotiline should not be taken with alcohol, sleeping pills, tranquilizers, or narcotic painkillers.

Recommended Dosage

Usual dosage for adults: 75 to 150 mg a day taken in one dose or several divided doses for mild to moderate depression; up to 225 mg a day for hospitalized patients suffering from moderate to severe depression.

Usual dosage for the elderly: 25 to 75 mg a day.

The safety and effectiveness of maprotiline use in children under eighteen years of age has not been established.

Overdosage

An overdose of maprotiline can be fatal. Symptoms of overdose may include agitation, bluish skin, convulsions, dilated pupils, drowsiness, fever, heart failure, involuntary writhing movements, irregular or rapid heartbeat, lack of coordination, loss of consciousness, low blood pressure, restlessness, rigid muscles, shock, and vomiting. If you experience any of these symptoms, go to the nearest hospital emergency room immediately.

Pregnancy and Lactation

The safety of maprotiline use during pregnancy has not been established. As a result, it should only be taken during pregnancy if the potential benefits clearly outweigh any potential risks to the fetus. If you are pregnant or plan to become pregnant, notify your doctor immediately.

The drug passes into breast milk and may be harmful to a nursing infant. Consequently, the drug should only be used by a nursing mother if the potential benefits of therapy clearly outweigh any potential risks to the infant.

Mesoridazine

Brand Name

Serentil

General Information

Mesoridazine is used in the treatment of psychotic disorders such as schizophrenia. It works by blocking the neurotransmitter dopamine. This suggests that many of the symptoms of psychosis may result from abnormal dopamine activity in the brain.

Symptoms of schizophrenia include delusions, hallucinations, disorganized speech, grossly disorganized or catatonic behavior, and absence of normal moods and emotions.

Side Effects

Mesoridazine may cause neuroleptic malignant syndrome (NMS), a rare but potentially life-threatening side effect characterized by severe muscle rigidity throughout the body. Other features of NMS include high fever, rapid heartbeat, rapid breathing, excessive perspiration, abnormal blood pressure, and kidney failure.

This drug also may cause a serious and at times permanent side effect called tardive dyskinesia. This neurological syndrome results in involuntary movements of the mouth, lips, and tongue such as tongue rolling, lip licking and smacking, chewing or sucking motions, pouting, and grimacing.

Other side effects may include abnormal contraction of the pupils; agitation; altered sex drive; anemia and other blood disorders; anorexia; asthma; bizarre dreams; blurred vision; breast development in males; complete or partial loss of muscle movement; constipation; contraction of the chewing muscles; defective muscular coordination; dermatitis; dizziness; drowsiness; dry mouth; edema; excitement; extreme constipation; fainting; false-positive pregnancy test; fever; impotence; inability to ejaculate; incontinence; involuntary fixation of the eyeballs; itching, jaundice; lactation; low blood pressure; menstrual irregularities; nausea; nipplelike growths on the tongue; paralysis of the intestines; Parkinson's syndrome; rapid heartbeat; rash; restlessness; rigidity; sensation of internal restlessness; severe and painful spasms of muscles in the head and neck; skin pigmentation; slurring; spasm in which the head and heels are bent backward and the body is bowed forward; stuffy nose; swelling of the larynx; tilting of the head to one side; tremors; unusual intolerance of light; urinary retention; vomiting; weakness; and weight gain.

If you experience any of these side effects or reactions, notify your doctor as soon as possible.

Important Precautions

Keep in mind that mesoridazine can cause neuroleptic malignant syndrome and tardive dyskinesia.

Do not take mesoridazine if you have ever had an allergic reaction or hypersensitivity to it or a similar drug.

Use this medication with caution if you have a history of breast cancer, low blood pressure, or seizures. Mesoridazine should also be used cautiously by people who are exposed to pesticides.

Mesoridazine may make you feel drowsy and impair your coordination. Do not drive, operate machinery, or participate in any high-risk activities until you know exactly how the drug affects you.

Food and Drug Interactions

If mesoridazine is taken with certain other drugs, the effects of either drug could be increased, decreased, or changed. Before beginning treatment with mesoridazine, tell your doctor if you are taking any other prescription or over-the-counter medications.

Mesoridazine should not be combined with alcohol, narcotics, sleeping pills, or tranquilizers.

Recommended Dosage

Usual dosage for adults: The usual starting dose is 50 mg three times a day. The optimum total daily dose typically ranges from 100 to 400 mg. Once symptoms are under control, it should be gradually lowered to the minimum effective dose.

The safety and effectiveness of mesoridazine use in children under the age of twelve has not been established.

Overdosage

An overdose of mesoridazine can be fatal. Symptoms of overdose may include accumulation of fluid in the tissues lining the larynx, agitation, blurred vision, cardiac abnormalities, cardiac arrest, coma, confusion, congestive heart failure, dilated pupils, disorientation, drowsiness, dry mouth, high fever, hyperactive reflexes, loss of reflexes, low blood pressure, nasal congestion, rapid heartbeat, rigid muscles, shock, spasms of the larynx, stupor, and vomiting. If you experience any of these symptoms, go to the nearest hospital emergency room immediately.

Pregnancy and Lactation

Mesoridazine should only be used during pregnancy if the potential benefits clearly outweigh any potential risks to the fetus. If you are pregnant or plan to become pregnant, notify your doctor immediately.

The drug may pass into breast milk and may be harmful to a nursing infant. If the medication is essential to your health, your doctor may advise you not to breast-feed while you are taking it.

Methylphenidate

Brand Name

Ritalin

General Information

Methylphenidate is a central nervous system stimulant used in the treatment of attention deficit disorder. It appears to work via effects on the neurotransmitter dopamine and/or the neurotransmitter norepinephrine.

Symptoms of attention deficit disorder include a chronic history of extreme distractibility, short attention span, physical or cognitive restlessness, impulsiveness, low tolerance for frustration, and mood swings.

This drug is also used to treat narcolepsy, a neurological condition characterized by an uncontrollable desire to sleep.

Side Effects

More common side effects may include insomnia and nervousness. In children, the more common side effects are abdominal pain, insomnia, loss of appetite, rapid heartbeat, and weight loss during long-term therapy.

Other side effects may include abnormal heartbeat; blood pressure changes; chest pain; dizziness; drowsiness; fever; headache; hives; jerking movements; joint pain; lack or loss of appetite; nausea; pounding heartbeat; pulse changes; rapid heartbeat; rash; reddish or purplish spots on the skin; skin inflammation and peeling; Tourette's syndrome (which is characterized by severe, multiple tics); uncontrollable twitching; weight loss during long-term therapy; and writhing movements.

If you experience any of these side effects or reactions, notify your doctor as soon as possible.

Important Precautions

Do not take methylphenidate if you have ever had an allergic reaction or hypersensitivity to it or a similar drug, or if you are anxious, tense, or agitated since the drug may intensify these symptoms.

Use this medication with caution if you have a

history of glaucoma, seizures, tics, or a family history of Tourette's syndrome. Caution should also be exercised when prescribing methylphenidate for emotionally unstable people, such as those suffering from alcoholism or drug dependence, because they may increase their dosage on their own.

Children should be carefully monitored during treatment with methylphenidate since growth suppression has been associated with long-term use of the drug.

Everyone taking methylphenidate, particularly those with hypertension, should have their blood pressure monitored regularly.

Food and Drug Interactions

If methylphenidate is taken with certain other drugs, the effects of either drug could be increased, decreased, or changed. Before beginning treatment with methylphenidate, tell your doctor if you are taking any other prescription or over-the-counter medications.

It is particularly important to check with your doctor before combining methylphenidate with anticonvulsants, blood thinners, monoamine oxidase inhibitors, tricyclic antidepressants, guanethidine (Ismelin), or phenylbutazone (Butazolidin).

Recommended Dosage

Usual dosage for adults: 20 to 30 mg a day taken in two or three divided doses, thirty to forty-five minutes before meals. Some people may need 40 to 60 mg a day; others may need only 10 to 15 mg a day. The dosage should be tailored to the individual.

Usual dosage for children: The usual starting dose is 5 mg taken twice a day, before breakfast and lunch. If necessary, this amount may gradually be increased in 5-to-10-mg increments until an effective dosage is reached. Dosages above 60 mg a day are not recommended.

Sustained-release tablets with an eight-hour action are also available.

The safety and effectiveness of methylphenidate use in children under the age of six has not been established.

Overdosage

Symptoms of a methylphenidate overdose may include agitation, confusion, convulsions, delirium, dryness of the mucous membranes, enlarged pupils, exaggerated feeling of elation, extremely high body temperature, flushing, hallucinations, headache, high blood pressure, irregular heartbeat, muscle twitching, palpitations, perspiration, rapid heartbeat, tremors, and vomiting. If you experience any of these symptoms, go to the nearest hospital emergency room immediately.

Pregnancy and Lactation

The safety of methylphenidate use during pregnancy has not been established. As a result, it should only be taken during pregnancy if the potential benefits clearly outweigh any potential risks to the fetus. If you are pregnant or plan to become pregnant, notify your doctor immediately.

The drug may pass into breast milk and may be harmful to a nursing infant. If the medication is

essential to your health, your doctor may advise you not to breast-feed while you are taking it.

Molindone

Brand Name
Moban

General Information
Molindone is used in the treatment of psychotic disorders such as schizophrenia. It works by blocking the neurotransmitter dopamine. This suggests that many of the symptoms of psychosis may result from abnormal dopamine activity in the brain.

Symptoms of schizophrenia include delusions, hallucinations, disorganized speech, grossly disorganized or catatonic behavior, and absence of normal moods and emotions.

Side Effects
Molindone may cause neuroleptic malignant syndrome (NMS), a rare but potentially life-threatening side effect characterized by severe muscle rigidity throughout the body. Other features of NMS include high fever, rapid heartbeat, rapid breathing, excessive perspiration, abnormal blood pressure, and kidney failure.

This drug also may cause a serious and at times permanent side effect called tardive dyskinesia. This neurological syndrome results in involuntary movements of the mouth, lips, and tongue such as tongue rolling, lip licking and smacking, chewing or sucking motions, pouting, and grimacing.

Other side effects may include absence of menstruation; blurred vision; breast development in males; constipation; depression; drowsiness; dry mouth; euphoria; hyperactivity; immobility; increased libido; nausea; rapid heartbeat; rash; reduction of voluntary movements; rigidity; salivation; sensation of internal restlessness; severe and painful spasms of muscles in the head and neck; spontaneous or excessive flow of milk; tremors; urinary retention; and weight gain or loss.

If you experience any of these side effects or reactions, notify your doctor as soon as possible.

Important Precautions

Keep in mind that molindone can cause neuroleptic malignant syndrome and tardive dyskinesia.

Do not take molindone if you have ever had an allergic reaction or hypersensitivity to it or a similar drug.

Use this medication with caution if you have a history of breast cancer, seizures, or hyperactivity.

Molindone may inhibit the vomiting reflex. As a result, it may mask the symptoms of drug overdose, brain tumors, intestinal blockage, and other conditions.

This drug may make you feel drowsy and impair your coordination. Do not drive, operate machinery, or participate in any high-risk activities until you know exactly how it affects you.

Food and Drug Interactions

If molindone is taken with certain other drugs, the effects of either drug could be increased, decreased, or changed. Before beginning treatment with molindone, tell your doctor if you are taking any other prescription or over-the-counter medications.

Molindone should not be combined with alcohol, narcotics, sleeping pills, or tranquilizers.

Recommended Dosage

Usual dosage for adults: The usual starting dose is 50 to 75 mg a day. If necessary, this amount may be increased to 100 mg a day over a three- or four-day period. An increase to 225 mg a day may be needed in patients with severe psychotic symptoms. Maintenance doses can range from as little as 15 mg a day to as much as 225 mg a day depending upon the severity of the psychotic symptoms.

Elderly and debilitated people should be started out on lower doses of molindone.

The safety and effectiveness of molindone use in children under the age of twelve has not been established.

Overdosage

Symptoms of a molindone overdose are usually the same as the side effects listed above. Some people, however, experience an intensification of these symptoms and/or additional symptoms such as stupor and coma. If you experience any of these symptoms, go to the nearest hospital emergency room immediately.

Pregnancy and Lactation

Molindone should only be taken during pregnancy if the potential benefits clearly outweigh any potential risks to the fetus. If you are pregnant or plan to become pregnant, notify your doctor immediately.

Studies have not determined the safety of using molindone during lactation. Consequently, the drug should only be used by a nursing mother if the potential benefits of therapy clearly outweigh any potential risks to the infant.

Nefazodone

Brand Name

Serzone

General Information

Nefazodone, which is used in the treatment of depression, is chemically unrelated to any other antidepressants on the market. It works by blocking the presynaptic reuptake of the neurotransmitters serotonin and norepinephrine in the brain. Nefazodone also blocks a class of serotonin receptors called S2 receptors. These facts suggest that many of the symptoms of depression may result from abnormalities in both serotonin and norepinephrine activity in the brain.

Symptoms of depression include low, anxious, or "empty" feelings; loss of interest and pleasure in activities previously enjoyed; noticeable change of appetite; noticeable change in sleeping patterns; fatigue or loss of energy; feelings of hopelessness or pessimism; feelings of guilt, worthlessness, or helplessness; inability to concentrate, make decisions, or remember details; recurring thoughts of death or suicide, wishing to die or attempting suicide; and aches and pains, constipation, or other physical ailments that cannot be explained.

Side Effects

More common side effects may include abnormal vision; blurred vision; bronchitis; confusion; constipation; difficulty breathing; dizziness; dry mouth; eye pain; impotence; inflammation of the stomach and intestinal tract; lack or loss of strength; lightheadedness; nausea; and sleepiness.

Less common side effects may include abnormal decrease of white blood cells; abnormal ejaculation; abnormal gait; abnormal liver function; abnormal sensitivity to sound; abnormal thinking; absence of menstruation; acne; anemia; apathy; arthritis; asthma; bad breath; belching; blood in the urine; breast enlargement; bursitis; chest pain; conjunctivitis; decreased attention; dehydration; difficult speech; dilated pupils; disease of the lymph nodes; double vision; dry eyes; dry skin; eczema; enlarged abdomen; euphoria; excessive menstrual bleeding; excessive urination; feelings of unreality; gout; hair loss; hallucinations; hangover effect; hernia; hiccups; high blood pressure; hostility; increased libido; inflammation of a tendon sheath, the bladder, colon, cornea and conjunctiva, esophagus, gums, mouth, stomach; intolerance of light; kidney stones; laryngitis; malaise; mouth ulceration; muscle stiffness, spasms, or twitching; nosebleed; paranoid reaction; pelvic pain; peptic ulcer; pneumonia; rapid heartbeat; rash; rectal bleeding; sense of detachment from one's surroundings; sensitivity to light; skin discoloration; suicidal thoughts; suicide; suicide attempt; swelling of the face; temporary loss of consciousness; tooth abscess; urinary incontinence; urinary urgency; uterine bleeding; vaginal bleeding; vertigo; voice alteration; and weight loss.

Rare side effects may include congestive heart failure; deafness; decreased urination; enlarged uterine fibroids; gastrointestinal bleeding; glaucoma; hemorrhage; hepatitis; high cholesterol; hyperventilation; inability to achieve orgasm; inability to swallow; increased muscular movement and physical activity; increased salivation; increased sensitivity to sensory stimuli; inflammation of the tongue; loss of muscle tone; loss of taste; low blood sugar; neuroleptic malignant syndrome; night blindness; oral infection; paleness; stroke; ulcerative colitis; yawning; and varicose veins.

If you experience any of these side effects or reactions, notify your doctor as soon as possible.

Important Precautions

Do not take nefazodone if you are taking another type of antidepressant called a monoamine oxidase inhibitor (MAOI) or have taken one within the past two weeks, or if you have ever had an allergic reaction or hypersensitivity to nefazodone or a similar drug.

Use this medication with caution if you have a

history of cardiovascular or liver disease, low blood pressure, mania, or seizures.

Nefazodone may impair your judgment, thinking, or motor skills. Do not drive, operate machinery, or participate in any high-risk activities until you know exactly how the drug affects you.

Discontinue the drug for as long as possible before undergoing elective surgery requiring anesthesia.

Notify your doctor if you develop a rash, hives, or a related allergic reaction while taking nefazodone.

Food and Drug Interactions

If nefazodone is taken with certain other drugs, the effects of either drug could be increased, decreased, or changed. Before beginning treatment with nefazodone, tell your doctor if you are taking any other prescription or over-the-counter medications.

Nefazodone should not be combined with MAOIs, astemizole (Hismanal), or terfenadine (Seldane). It is also important to check with your doctor before combining nefazodone with alprazolam (Xanax), digoxin (Lanoxin), haloperidol (Haldol), triazolam (Halcion), or drugs that are active in the central nervous system.

Do not drink alcohol while taking nefazodone.

Recommended Dosage

Usual dosage for adults: The usual starting dose is 100 mg twice a day. This amount may be increased to 150 mg twice a day after one week. Effective dosages range from 300 to 600 mg a day.

Usual dosage for the elderly: The usual starting dose is 50 mg twice a day.

The safety and effectiveness of nefazodone use in children under the age of eighteen has not been established.

Overdosage

Symptoms of a nefazodone overdose may include nausea, sleepiness, and vomiting. If you experience any of these symptoms, go to the nearest hospital emergency room immediately.

Pregnancy and Lactation

The safety of nefazodone use during pregnancy has not been established. As a result, it should only be taken during pregnancy if the potential benefits clearly outweigh any potential risks to the fetus. If you are pregnant or plan to become pregnant, notify your doctor immediately.

Studies have also not determined the safety of using nefazodone during lactation. Consequently, the drug should only be used by a nursing mother if the potential benefits of therapy clearly outweigh any potential risks to the infant.

Nortriptyline

Brand Name

Pamelor

General Information

Nortriptyline is used to treat depression. It is a member of the class of drugs called tricyclic antidepressants, which work by blocking the presynaptic reuptake of the neurotransmitters serotonin, norepinephrine, and dopamine in the brain. This suggests that many of the symptoms of depression may result from imbalances of one or more of these neurotransmitters.

Symptoms of depression include low, anxious, or "empty" feelings; loss of interest and pleasure in activities previously enjoyed; noticeable change of appetite; noticeable change in sleeping patterns; fatigue or loss of energy; feelings of hopelessness or pessimism; feelings of guilt, worthlessness, or helplessness; inability to concentrate, make decisions, or remember details; recurring thoughts of death or suicide, wishing to die or attempting suicide; and aches and pains, constipation, or other physical ailments that cannot be explained.

Side Effects

Side effects may include abdominal cramps; agitation; anxiety; black tongue; blurred vision; breast development in males; breast enlargement; confusion; constipation; diarrhea; dilated pupils; disorientation;

dizziness; drowsiness; dry mouth; excessive or spontaneous flow of milk; excessive urination at night; fatigue; fluid retention; flushing; frequent urination or difficulty or delay in urinating; hair loss; hallucinations; headache; heart attack; high or low blood pressure; high or low blood sugar; hives; impotence; increased or decreased sex drive; inflammation of the mouth; insomnia; intestinal blockage; itching; loss of appetite; loss of coordination; nausea; nightmares; numbness; odd taste in mouth; panic; perspiration; rapid, pounding, or irregular heartbeat; rash; reddish or purplish spots on the skin; restlessness; ringing in the ears; sensitivity to light; stomach upset; stroke; swelling of the testicles; tingling; tremors; vomiting; weakness; weight gain or loss; and yellowed skin and whites of eyes.

If you experience any of these side effects or reactions, notify your doctor as soon as possible.

Important Precautions

Do not take nortriptyline if you have had a heart attack recently, if you are taking another type of antidepressant called a monoamine oxidase inhibitor (MAOI) or have taken one within the past two weeks, if you are taking any other antidepressants, or if you have ever had an allergic reaction or hypersensitivity to nortriptyline or a similar drug.

Use this medication with caution if you are being treated for a severe mental illness such as schizophrenia or manic depression or if you have a history of cardiovascular or thyroid disease, glaucoma or other chronic eye conditions, seizures, or urinary retention.

Nortriptyline may make you feel dizzy and drowsy. Do not drive, operate machinery, or participate in any high-risk activities until you know exactly how the drug affects you.

Abruptly discontinuing nortriptyline may result in headaches, nausea, and other unpleasant side effects. When ending treatment with this drug, follow your doctor's schedule for a gradual withdrawal.

Be sure to inform your doctor or dentist that you are taking nortriptyline before undergoing any type of surgery or dental treatment.

Food and Drug Interactions

If nortriptyline is taken with certain other drugs, the effects of either drug could be increased, decreased, or changed. Before beginning treatment with nortriptyline, tell your doctor if you are taking any other prescription or over-the-counter medications.

Combining nortriptyline with a MAOI can lead to extremely high fever, severe convulsions, even death. If you have been taking a MAOI, you must wait at least two weeks after discontinuing therapy with the drug before starting therapy with nortriptyline.

It is also important to check with your doctor before combining nortriptyline with sedative or hypnotic drugs, muscle relaxants, thyroid medications, albuterol (Proventil, Ventolin), cimetidine (Tagamet), fluoxetine (Prozac), or guanethidine (Ismelin).

Nortriptyline should not be taken with alcohol, sleeping pills, tranquilizers, or narcotic painkillers.

Recommended Dosage

Usual dosage for adults: The usual starting dosage is 75 to 100 mg a day taken in one dose or several divided doses.

Usual dosage for adolescents and the elderly: The usual starting dosage is 30 to 50 mg a day taken in one dose or two divided doses.

Dosages above 150 mg a day are not recommended. Nortriptyline is not recommended for children.

Overdosage

An overdose of nortriptyline can be fatal. Symptoms of overdose may include agitation, coma, confusion, congestive heart failure, convulsions, decreased breathing, excessive reflexes, extremely high fever, rapid heartbeat, restlessness, rigid muscles, shock, stupor, and vomiting. If you experience any of these symptoms, go to the nearest hospital emergency room immediately.

Pregnancy and Lactation

The safety of nortriptyline use during pregnancy has not been established. As a result, it should only be taken during pregnancy if the potential benefits clearly outweigh any potential risks to the fetus. If you are pregnant or plan to become pregnant, notify your doctor immediately.

Studies have also not determined the safety of using nortriptyline during lactation. Consequently, the drug should only be used by a nursing mother if the potential benefits of therapy clearly outweigh any potential risks to the infant.

Oxazepam

Brand Names

Serax

General Information

Oxazepam is used in the short-term treatment of anxiety disorder, panic disorder, and anxiety associated with depression. It is also used to relieve the symptoms of alcohol withdrawal. It is a member of the class of drugs called benzodiazepines, which facilitate the action of the neurotransmitter GABA (gamma-aminobutyric acid). At lower doses, oxazepam decreases anxiety. At higher doses, it causes sedation and sleep. Oxazepam relaxes skeletal muscles as well.

Symptoms of anxiety include trembling, twitching, heart palpitations, shortness of breath, sweaty palms, clammy skin, dry mouth, dizziness, nausea, and trouble swallowing.

Side Effects

A more common side effect is drowsiness.

Less common or rare side effects may include blood disorders; change in sex drive; dizziness; double or blurred vision; euphoria; fever; hallucinations; headache; lack or loss or muscle control; loss of urinary control; menstrual irregularities; nausea; rage; rash; sluggishness or unresponsiveness; slurred speech; spastic muscles; stimulation; swelling due to fluid retention; and tremors.

If you experience any of these side effects or reactions, notify your doctor as soon as possible.

Important Precautions

Do not take oxazepam if you are being treated for a mental illness more severe than anxiety or if you have ever had an allergic reaction or hypersensitivity to oxazepam or a similar drug.

Use this medication with caution if you have a history of liver, kidney, or heart disease.

Oxazepam may make you drowsy or less alert. Do not drive, operate machinery, or participate in any high-risk activities until you know exactly how the drug affects you.

Some people, especially those who are allergic to aspirin, have experienced an allergic reaction to the yellow food coloring contained in oxazepam.

Abruptly discontinuing oxazepam may result in withdrawal symptoms such as abdominal and muscle cramps, convulsions, depressed mood, insomnia, perspiration, tremors, and vomiting. When ending treatment with this medication, follow your doctor's schedule for a gradual withdrawal.

Food and Drug Interactions

If oxazepam is taken with certain other drugs, the effects of either drug could be increased, decreased, or changed. Before beginning treatment with oxazepam, tell your doctor if you are taking any other prescription or over-the-counter medications.

It is particularly important to check with your doctor before combining oxazepam with antihistamines and other central nervous system depressants.

Do not drink alcohol while taking oxazepam.

Recommended Dosage

Usual dosage for adults: The usual starting dosage is 10 to 15 mg three or four times a day. For severe anxiety, this amount may be increased to 15 to 30 mg three or four times a day.

Usual dosage for the elderly: The usual starting dose is 10 mg three times a day. If necessary, this amount may be increased to 15 mg three or four times a day.

Oxazepam should not be used by children under the age of six. Dosages for children between the ages of six and twelve have not been established.

Overdosage

Symptoms of an oxazepam overdose may include coma, confusion, sleepiness, and slowed reflexes. If you experience any of these symptoms, go to the nearest hospital emergency room immediately.

Pregnancy and Lactation

Oxazepam may cause birth defects. As a result, it should not be taken during pregnancy. If you are pregnant or plan to become pregnant, notify your doctor immediately.

The drug may pass into breast milk and may be harmful to a nursing infant. If the medication is essential to your health, your doctor may advise you not to breast-feed while you are taking it.

Paroxetine

Brand Name
Paxil

General Information

Paroxetine is used to treat depression. It is a member of the class of drugs called selective serotonin reuptake inhibitors, which work by blocking the presynaptic reuptake of the neurotransmitter serotonin. This suggests that many of the symptoms of depression may result from abnormal serotonin activity in the brain.

Symptoms of depression include low, anxious, or "empty" feelings; loss of interest and pleasure in activities previously enjoyed; noticeable change of appetite; noticeable change in sleeping patterns; fatigue or loss of energy; feelings of hopelessness or pessimism; feelings of guilt, worthlessness, or helplessness; inability to concentrate, make decisions, or remember details; recurring thoughts of death or suicide, wishing to die or attempting suicide; and aches and pains, constipation, or other physical ailments that cannot be explained.

Side Effects

More common side effects may include abnormal ejaculation and other male genital disorders; agitation; amnesia; anxiety; central nervous system stimulation; chills; decreased appetite; depression; diarrhea; dizziness; dry mouth; emotional swings; hypertension; impaired concentration; increased cough; insomnia; lack or loss of strength; malaise; nausea; rapid heartbeat; rhinitis; severe itching; sleepiness; sweating; swelling due to fluid retention; temporary loss of consciousness; tremors; vertigo; vomiting; and weight gain or loss.

Less common side effects may include abnormal decrease of white blood cells; abnormal electrocardiogram; abnormal liver function tests; abnormal tension of arteries or muscles; abnormal thinking; absence of menstruation; acne; alcohol abuse; anemia; arthritis; asthma; belching; boils; breast pain; bronchitis; cancer; complete or partial loss of muscle movement; convulsions; defective muscular coordination; difficulty breathing; difficulty swallowing; dilated pupils; disease of the arteries and veins of the extremities; disease of the lymph nodes; dry skin; ear pain; eczema; excessive menstrual bleeding; excessive urination during the night; eye pain; facial swelling; feelings of unreality; grinding of the teeth; hair loss; hallucinations; high blood sugar; hyperventilation; increased muscular movement and physical activity; increased salivation; infection of the skin or mucous membranes; inflammation of the bladder, sinuses, stomach, tongue, or urethra; joint pain; lack of coordination; lack of emotion; loss of taste; low blood pressure; mania; migraine; miscarriage; mouth ulceration; neck pain; nosebleed; painful menstruation; painful or difficult urination; pneumonia; rash; rectal bleeding; respiratory flu; ringing in the ears; skin discoloration; slow heartbeat; swelling of the extremities; thirst; urinary incontinence; urinary retention; urinary urgency; and vaginitis.

Rare side effects may include abnormal gait; abnormal kidney function; abnormal protrusion of the eyes;

abnormal sensitivity to sound; abnormally low calcium; abscesses; anemia; antisocial reaction; black stool; bleeding from the eyes; blood clot; blood in the urine; bloody diarrhea; breast cancer; breast tumors; bulimia; bursitis; cataracts; chest pain; congestive heart failure; conjunctivitis; decreased motor reaction to stimulus; defect in voluntary movement; dehydration; delirium; delusions; diabetes mellitus; difficult speech; disease of the nerves; double vision; drug dependence; euphoria; excess of lymph cells; excessive sensitivity to pain; extremely low potassium; fecal impactions; fecal incontinence; formation of scar tissue in the lungs; glaucoma; gout; grand mal seizure; hepatitis; hiccups; high cholesterol; hostility; hyperthyroidism; hypothyroidism; hysteria; increased reflexes; increased sex drive; increased sputum; inflammation of bone marrow, muscle tissue, vein, breasts, colon, ear, esophagus, first part of the small intestine, gums, kidney, skin, stomach and intestinal tract; thyroid; intestinal blockage; involuntary eyeball movement; jaundice; jerky involuntary movements; joint disease; kidney pain; kidney stones; lactation in women; low blood sugar; low cardiac output; low sodium; lung cancer; manic depression; meningitis; neck rigidity; osteoporosis; paleness; paralysis; pelvic pain; peptic ulcer; prolonged muscle contractions; prostate cancer; psychosis; psychotic depression; rash; red and painful nodules on the legs; reduction of breast size; reduction or dimness of vision; salivary gland enlargement; severe pain along the course of a nerve; skin cancer; skin discoloration; stomach ulcer; stroke; stupor; swelling of the tongue; temporary deficiency in blood supply to the brain; tooth decay; ulceration of the cornea; unusual intolerance of light; urinary deficiency; vaginal infection; varicose veins;

vascular headache; vomiting of blood; and withdrawal syndrome.

If you experience any of these side effects or reactions, notify your doctor as soon as possible.

Important Precautions

Serious, sometimes fatal, reactions have resulted from taking paroxetine with another type of antidepressant called a monoamine oxidase inhibitor (MAOI), and when paroxetine therapy is discontinued and MAOI therapy is started. Never take paroxetine with one of these drugs or within two weeks of ending treatment with one of these drugs.

Do not take paroxetine if you have ever had an allergic reaction or hypersensitivity to it or a similar drug.

Use this medication with caution if you have a history of kidney or liver disease, mania, or seizures.

Paroxetine may make you feel dizzy and drowsy. Do not drive, operate machinery, or participate in any high-risk activities until you know exactly how the drug affects you.

Food and Drug Interactions

If paroxetine is taken with certain other drugs, the effects of either drug could be increased, decreased, or changed. Before beginning treatment with paroxetine, tell your doctor if you are taking any other prescription or over-the-counter medications.

Paroxetine should not be combined with MAOIs or the amino acid tryptophan. It is also important to check with your doctor before combining paroxetine with cimetidine (Tagamet), digoxin (Lanoxin), lithium (Eskalith, Lithobid), phenobarbital, phenytoin (Dilantin), procyclidine, warfarin (Coumadin), other antidepressants, antiarrythmic drugs, and antipsychotic drugs known as phenothiazines.

Do not drink alcohol while taking paroxetine.

Recommended Dosage

Usual dosage for adults: The usual starting dose is 20 mg a day taken in the morning. If necessary, this amount may gradually be increased by 10-mg increments to a maximum of 50 mg a day.

Usual dosage for the elderly: The usual starting dose is 10 mg a day. Dosages above 40 mg a day are not recommended.

The safety and effectiveness of paroxetine use in children has not been established.

Overdosage

Symptoms of a paroxetine overdose may include dilated pupils, drowsiness, nausea, and vomiting. If you experience any of these symptoms, go to the nearest hospital emergency room immediately.

Pregnancy and Lactation

The safety of paroxetine use during pregnancy has not been established. If you are pregnant or plan to become pregnant, notify your doctor immediately.

Paroxetine passes into breast milk and may be harmful to a nursing infant. If the medication is essential to your health, your doctor may advise you not to breast-feed while you are taking it.

Pemoline

Brand Name
Cylert

General Information

Pemoline is a central nervous system stimulant used in the treatment of attention deficit disorder. It appears to work via effects on the neurotransmitters dopamine and/or norepinephrine.

Symptoms of attention deficit disorder include a chronic history of extreme distractibility, short attention span, physical or cognitive restlessness, impulsiveness, low tolerance for frustration, and mood swings.

This drug is also used to treat narcolepsy, a neurological condition characterized by an uncontrollable desire to sleep.

Side Effects

A more common side effect is insomnia.

Other side effects may include dizziness; drowsiness; hallucinations; headache; increased irritability; involuntary movements of the face, eyes, lips, tongue, arms, and legs; liver problems; loss of appetite; mild depression; nausea; rash; seizures; stomachache; suppressed growth in children; uncontrolled vocal outbursts (such as shouts, grunts, and obscene language); weight loss; and yellowing of the skin or whites of the eyes.

Rare side effects may include a rare form of anemia

accompanied by bleeding gums, bruising, chest pain, fatigue, headache, nosebleeds, and pallor.

If you experience any of these side effects or reactions, notify your doctor as soon as possible.

Important Precautions

Do not take pemoline if you have liver problems or if you have ever had an allergic reaction or hypersensitivity to pemoline or a similar drug.

Use this medication with caution if you have a history of kidney problems or alcohol or drug abuse.

Pemoline may make you feel dizzy. Do not drive, operate machinery, or participate in any high-risk activities until you know exactly how the drug affects you.

Children should be carefully monitored during treatment with pemoline since growth suppression has been associated with long-term use of the drug.

Food and Drug Interactions

If pemoline is taken with certain other drugs, the effects of either drug could be increased, decreased, or changed. Before beginning treatment with pemoline, tell your doctor if you are taking any other prescription or over-the-counter medications.

It is particularly important to check with your doctor before combining pemoline with anticonvulsants or other drugs that act on the central nervous system.

Recommended Dosage

Usual dosage for children: The usual starting dose is 37.5 mg a day. If necessary, this amount may be increased by 18.75 mg at one-week intervals until the optimum therapeutic benefit is achieved. Most children take doses ranging from 56.25 mg to 75 mg a day. Dosages above 112.5 mg are not recommended.

For adults other than the elderly, higher doses may be needed.

Dosages for the elderly should be individually tailored by a doctor.

Overdosage

Symptoms of a pemoline overdose may include agitation; coma; confusion; convulsions; delirium; dilated pupils; euphoria; extremely high body temperature; flushing; hallucinations; headache; high blood pressure; increased heart rate; increased reflex reactions; muscle twitching; perspiration; tremors; and vomiting. If you experience any of these symptoms, go to the nearest hospital emergency room immediately.

Pregnancy and Lactation

Pemoline should only be taken during pregnancy if the potential benefits clearly outweigh any potential risks to the fetus. If you are pregnant or plan to become pregnant, notify your doctor immediately.

The drug may pass into breast milk and may be harmful to a nursing infant. If the medication is essential to your health, your doctor may advise you not to breast-feed while you are taking it.

Perphenazine

Brand Name
Trilafon

General Information
Perphenazine is used in the treatment of psychotic disorders such as schizophrenia. It works by blocking the neurotransmitter dopamine. This suggests that many of the symptoms of psychosis may result from abnormal dopamine activity in the brain.

Symptoms of schizophrenia include delusions, hallucinations, disorganized speech, grossly disorganized or catatonic behavior, and absence of normal moods and emotions.

Side Effects
Perphenazine may cause neuroleptic malignant syndrome (NMS), a rare but potentially life-threatening side effect characterized by severe muscle rigidity throughout the body. Other features of NMS include high fever, rapid heartbeat, rapid breathing, excessive perspiration, abnormal blood pressure, and kidney failure.

This drug also may cause a serious and at times permanent side effect called tardive dyskinesia. This neurological syndrome results in involuntary movements of the mouth, lips, and tongue such as tongue rolling, lip licking and smacking, chewing or sucking motions, pouting, and grimacing.

Other side effects may include abnormal gait; aching and numbness of the limbs; anorexia; asthma; bizarre dreams; bladder paralysis; blood disorders; blurred vision; breast development in males; cardiac arrest; catatonic-like state; change in pulse rate; constipation; contraction of the muscles used in chewing; convulsive seizures; defect in voluntary movement; defective muscular coordination; diarrhea; dilated pupils; dizziness; dry mouth; eating abnormally large amounts of food at a meal; eczema; excessive flow of milk; excitement; fainting; false-positive pregnancy tests; fever; glaucoma; head tilting to one side; headache; high blood pressure; high blood sugar; hyperactivity; inability to ejaculate; inability to swallow or difficulty in swallowing; increase in appetite and weight; increased or decreased sex drive; increased reflexes; insomnia; intestinal blockage; involuntary fixation of the eyeballs; lactation; lethargy; liver damage; low blood pressure; low blood sugar; menstrual-cycle disturbances; moderate breast enlargement in females; motor restlessness; muscle weakness and rigidity; nasal congestion; nausea; nighttime confusion; paleness; paranoid reaction; perspiration; protrusion, discoloration, aching, and rounding of the tongue; rapid heartbeat; red, itchy, scaly skin; salivation; severe itching; skin pigmentation; slow heartbeat; slurred speech; spasm in which the head and heels are bent backward and the body is bowed forward; spasm of the muscles in the back of the neck; sugar in the urine; swelling of brain tissue, extremities, or larynx; tight feeling in the throat; unusual intolerance of light; urinary retention, frequency, or incontinence; vision changes; vomiting; worsening of psychotic symptoms; and yellowing of the skin and whites of the eyes.

If you experience any of these side effects or reactions, notify your doctor as soon as possible.

Important Precautions

Keep in mind that perphenazine can cause neuroleptic malignant syndrome and tardive dyskinesia.

Do not take perphenazine if you have a blood disease, bone-marrow depression, liver damage, or subcortical brain damage, or if you have ever had an allergic reaction or hypersensitivity to perphenazine or a similar drug.

Use this medication with caution if you have a history of breast cancer, liver disease, psychic depression, seizures, reduced kidney function, respiratory impairment, or pheochromocytoma (a small tumor of the adrenal gland). Perphenazine should also be used cautiously by people who are exposed to extreme heat or insecticides as well as those who are taking diarrhea medications.

Perphenazine may inhibit the vomiting reflex. As a result, it may mask the symptoms of drug overdose, brain tumors, intestinal blockage, and other conditions.

This drug may make you feel drowsy and impair your coordination. Do not drive, operate machinery, or participate in any high-risk activities until you know exactly how it affects you.

Since perphenazine can make you sensitive to light, try to stay out of the sun as much as possible during treatment.

Abruptly discontinuing perphenazine may result in dizziness, gastritis, nausea, trembling, and vomiting. When ending treatment with this medication, follow your doctor's schedule for a gradual withdrawal.

Food and Drug Interactions

If perphenazine is taken with certain other drugs, the effects of either drug could be increased, decreased, or changed. Before beginning treatment with perphenazine, tell your doctor if you are taking any other prescription or over-the-counter medications.

Perphenazine should not be combined with alcohol, narcotics, sleeping pills, or tranquilizers.

Recommended Dosage

Usual dosage for adults: The usual starting dose is 50 to 75 mg a day. If necessary, this amount may be increased to 100 mg a day over a three- or four-day period. An increase to 225 mg a day may be needed for patients with severe psychotic symptoms. Maintenance doses can range from as little as 15 mg a day to as much as 225 mg a day depending upon the severity of the psychotic symptoms.

Elderly and debilitated people should be started out on lower doses of perphenazine.

The safety and effectiveness of perphenazine use in children under the age of twelve has not been established.

Overdosage

Symptoms of a perphenazine overdose are usually the same as the side effects listed above. Some people, however, experience an intensification of these symptoms and/or additional symptoms such as stupor and coma. If you experience any of these symptoms, go to the nearest hospital emergency room immediately.

Pregnancy and Lactation

The safety of perphenazine use during pregnancy has not been established. As a result, it should only be taken during pregnancy if the potential benefits clearly outweigh any potential risks to the fetus. If you are pregnant or plan to become pregnant, notify your doctor immediately.

Studies have also not determined the safety of using perphenazine during lactation. Consequently, the drug should only be used by a nursing mother if the potential benefits of therapy clearly outweigh any potential risks to the infant.

Phenelzine

Brand Name

Nardil

General Information

Phenelzine is used to treat depression and anxiety as well as panic disorder and phobias mixed with depression. It is a member of the class of drugs called monoamine oxidase inhibitors (MAOIs). Monoamine oxidase is an enzyme that breaks down the neurotransmitters serotonin, norepinephrine, and dopamine. Phenelzine helps to create more balanced moods by blocking the effects of monoamine oxidase. Unfortunately, blocking monoamine oxidase throughout the entire body can cause serious side effects if a patient is not scrupulously careful about avoiding certain foods and medications. For this reason, MAOIs are typically reserved for situations in which other antidepressant drug treatments have failed.

Symptoms of depression include low, anxious, or "empty" feelings; loss of interest and pleasure in activities previously enjoyed; noticeable change of appetite; noticeable change in sleeping patterns; fatigue or loss of energy; feelings of hopelessness or pessimism; feelings of guilt, worthlessness, or helplessness; inability to concentrate, make decisions, or remember details; recurring thoughts of death or suicide, wishing to die or attempting suicide; and aches and pains, constipation, or other physical ailments that cannot be explained.

Side Effects

Common side effects may include constipation; disorders of the stomach and intestines; dizziness; drowsiness; dry mouth; excessive sleeping; fatigue; headache; insomnia; low blood pressure; muscle spasms; sexual difficulties; swelling due to fluid retention; tremors; twitching; weakness; and weight gain.

Less common or rare side effects may include anxiety; blurred vision; coma; convulsions; euphoria; fever; glaucoma; lack of coordination; liver damage; mania; nervousness; onset of schizophrenia; perspiration; rapid breathing; rapid eye movements; rapid heart rate; rash; rigid muscles; speech disorders; swelling in the throat; tingling sensation; urinary difficulties; and yellowed skin and whites of the eyes.

If you experience any of these side effects or reactions, notify your doctor as soon as possible.

Important Precautions

Taking phenelzine with certain foods, beverages, and medications can cause serious, potentially fatal, high blood pressure. For detailed information on substances to avoid, see the "Food and Drug Interactions" section below.

Do not take phenelzine if you have pheochromocytoma (a small tumor of the adrenal gland), congestive heart failure, a history of liver disease, or if you have ever had an allergic reaction or hypersensitivity to phenelzine or a similar drug.

Use this medication with caution if you have diabetes since scientists do not yet know how MAOIs affect blood sugar levels.

Be sure to inform your doctor or dentist that you are taking phenelzine, or have taken it within the past two weeks, before having any type of surgery or dental treatment. Do not undergo elective surgery requiring anesthesia while you are on the drug. Always carry a card or wear a bracelet that says you take phenelzine.

On rare occasions, abruptly discontinuing phenelzine results in convulsions, nightmares, strange behavior, and other unpleasant side effects.

Food and Drug Interactions

If phenelzine is taken with certain other drugs, the effects of either drug could be increased, decreased, or changed. Before beginning treatment with phenelzine, tell your doctor if you are taking any other prescription or over-the-counter medications.

The use of any MAOI requires patients to observe rigid dietary restrictions since foods containing a naturally occurring substance called tyramine can interact with the drug and trigger a sudden, potentially life-threatening rise in blood pressure. Foods to avoid while taking phenelzine, and for two weeks after discontinuing treatment with the medication, include beer (including alcohol-free or reduced-alcohol brands); caffeine (in excessive amounts); cheese (except for cottage cheese and cream cheese); dry sausage (including salami and pepperoni); fava beans; liver; meat extract; pickled, fermented, aged, or smoked meat, fish, or dairy products; pickled herring; sauerkraut; wine (including alcohol-free and reduced-alcohol brands); yeast extract (including large amounts of brewer's yeast); and yogurt.

A number of prescription and over-the-counter drugs must be avoided as well, including amphetamines, appetite suppressants, asthma inhalants, central nervous system stimulants, cold and cough preparations, hay fever medications, nasal decongestants, other antidepressants, products containing L-tryptophan, and sinus medications. For a complete list of prohibited foods, beverages, and medications, see your doctor.

Blood pressure medications should also be used with caution when taking phenelzine since they may lead to abnormally low pressure. Symptoms of low blood pressure include dizziness when rising from a seated or prone position, fainting, and tingling in the hands or feet. If you experience any of these symptoms, or any other unusual symptoms, inform your doctor immediately.

Phenelzine should not be taken with alcohol.

Recommended Dosage

Usual dosage for adults: The usual starting dose is 15 mg three times a day. If necessary, this amount may be increased to 90 mg a day. Once the maximum therapeutic benefit has been reached, the dosage may gradually be lowered. Maintenance doses of 15 mg a day or every two days are not unusual.

The safety and effectiveness of phenelzine use in children under the age of sixteen has not been established.

Overdosage

An overdose of phenelzine can be fatal. Symptoms of overdose may include agitation; backward arching of the head, neck, and back; coma; convulsions; cool, clammy skin; difficulty breathing; dizziness, drowsiness; faintness; hallucinations; high fever; high or low blood pressure; hyperactivity; irritability; jaw-muscle spasms; pain in the heart area; perspiration; rapid and irregular pulse; and severe headache. If you experience any of these symptoms, go to the nearest hospital emergency room immediately.

Pregnancy and Lactation

The safety of phenelzine use during pregnancy has not been established. As a result, it should only be taken during pregnancy if the potential benefits clearly outweigh any potential risks to the fetus. If you are pregnant or plan to become pregnant, notify your doctor immediately.

Studies have also not determined the safety of using phenelzine during lactation. Consequently, the drug should only be used by a nursing mother if the potential benefits of therapy clearly outweigh any potential risks to the infant.

Pimozide

Brand Name
Orap

General Information

Pimozide is used in the treatment of severe Tourette's syndrome. It is also sometimes prescribed for the treatment of schizophrenia, although it has not been approved by the FDA for this purpose. It works by blocking the neurotransmitter dopamine. This suggests that many of the symptoms of schizophrenia may result from abnormal dopamine activity in the brain.

Symptoms of schizophrenia include delusions, hallucinations, disorganized speech, grossly disorganized or catatonic behavior, and absence of normal moods and emotions.

Side Effects

Pimozide may cause neuroleptic malignant syndrome (NMS), a rare but potentially life-threatening side effect characterized by severe muscle rigidity throughout the body. Other features of NMS include high fever, rapid heartbeat, rapid breathing, excessive perspiration, abnormal blood pressure, and kidney failure.

This drug may also cause a serious and at times permanent side effect called tardive dyskinesia. This neurological syndrome results in involuntary movements of the mouth, lips, and tongue such as tongue rolling, lip licking and smacking, chewing or sucking motions, pouting, and grimacing.

Other side effects may include altered mental state; behavioral changes; belching; blood pressure changes; blurred vision; changes in heart rhythm; chewing movements; constant trembling of the hands; constipation; diarrhea; dizziness; drooling; drowsiness; dry mouth; excessive thirst; fine, wormlike movement of the tongue; handwriting change; headache; impotence; inability to sit still; increased appetite; increased body temperature; involuntary movements of the tongue, face, mouth, or jaw; irregular pulse; lightheadedness; loss of movement; loss of sex drive; muscular weakness and rigidity; nausea; pounding in the chest; protrusion of the tongue; puckering of the mouth; puffing of the cheeks; rash; rigid stoop; sedation; speech disorders; stiff, shuffling walk; stiffness; stomach upset; sweating; swelling around the eyes; tremors; unblinking, fixed gaze; uncontrollable jerking or twitching; visual problems; vomiting; and weakness.

If you experience any of these side effects or reactions, notify your doctor as soon as possible.

Important Precautions

Keep in mind that pimozide can cause neuroleptic malignant syndrome and tardive dyskinesia.

Do not take pimozide if you have ever had an allergic reaction or sensitivity to it or to any other antipsychotic drug.

This drug may also not be appropriate for people who have a history of abnormal heart rhythm or simple tics, or who are taking medications that may cause tics such as dextroamphetamine (Dexedrine), methylphenidate (Ritalin), and pemoline (Cylert).

Pimozide may make you drowsy. Do not drive, operate machinery, or participate in any high-risk activities until you know exactly how the drug affects you.

Food and Drug Interactions

If pimozide is taken with certain other drugs, the effects of either drug could be increased, decreased, or changed. Before beginning treatment with pimozide, tell your doctor if you are taking any other prescription or over-the-counter medications.

It is particularly important to check with your doctor before taking pimozide with anticonvulsants, antiarrhythmic drugs, central nervous system depressants, other antipsychotic drugs or tricyclic antidepressants.

Avoid drinking alcoholic beverages while taking pimozide.

Recommended Dosage

Usual dosage for adults: The usual starting dose is 1 to 2 mg a day taken in divided doses. If necessary, this amount may gradually be increased until an effective dose is reached. Dosages above 20 mg a day are not recommended.

Lower dosages are recommended for children and the elderly.

Overdosage

An overdose of pimozide can be fatal. Symptoms of a pimozide overdose may include coma, irregular heartbeat, low blood pressure, severe involuntary movements, and slowed breathing. If you experience any of these symptoms, go to the nearest hospital emergency room immediately.

Pregnancy and Lactation

Pimozide should only be used during pregnancy if the potential benefits clearly outweigh any potential risks to the fetus. If you are pregnant or plan to become pregnant, notify your doctor immediately.

The drug may pass into breast milk and may be harmful to a nursing infant. If the medication is essential to your health, your doctor may advise you not to breast-feed while you are taking it.

Prazepam

Brand Name
Centrax

General Information
Prazepam is used in the treatment of anxiety disorders. It is a member of the class of drugs called benzodiazepines, which facilitate the action of the neurotransmitter GABA (gamma-aminobutyric acid). At lower doses, prazepam decreases anxiety. At higher doses, it causes sedation and sleep. Prazepam relaxes skeletal muscles as well.

Symptoms of anxiety include trembling, twitching, heart palpitations, shortness of breath, sweaty palms, clammy skin, dry mouth, dizziness, nausea, and trouble swallowing.

Side Effects
More common side effects may include dizziness, drowsiness, fatigue, lack of muscular coordination, light-headedness, and weakness.

Less common or rare side effects may include blurred vision; confusion; dry mouth; excessive perspiration; fainting; genital and urinary tract disorders; headache; itching; joint pain; palpitations; rash; slurred speech; stomach and intestinal disorders; swelling of the feet; tremors; and vivid dreams.

If you experience any of these side effects or reactions, notify your doctor as soon as possible.

Important Precautions

Do not take prazepam if you have acute narrow-angle glaucoma, if you are being treated for a mental illness more severe than anxiety, or if you have ever had an allergic reaction or hypersensitivity to prazepam or a similar drug.

Use this medication with caution if you are severely depressed or if you have a history of severe depression.

Prazepam may make you drowsy or less alert. Do not drive, operate machinery, or participate in any high-risk activities until you know exactly how the drug affects you.

Abruptly discontinuing prazepam may result in withdrawal symptoms such as abdominal and muscle cramps, convulsions, tremors, and vomiting. When ending treatment with this medication, follow your doctor's schedule for a gradual withdrawal.

Food and Drug Interactions

If prazepam is taken with certain other drugs, the effects of either drug could be increased, decreased, or changed. Before beginning treatment with prazepam, tell your doctor if you are taking any other prescription or over-the-counter medications.

It is particularly important to check with your doctor before combining prazepam with antidepressants and other central nervous system depressants including barbiturates, monoamine oxidase inhibitors, narcotics, chlorpromazine (Thorazine), and promethazine (Phenergan).

Do not drink alcohol while taking prazepam.

Recommended Dosage

Usual dosage for adults: The usual starting dosage is 30 mg a day taken in several divided doses. Some people may only need 20 mg a day; others may need up to 60 mg a day. The dosage should be tailored to the individual. Prazepam may also be taken in a single dose at bedtime.

Usual dosage for the elderly: The usual starting dosage is 10 to 15 mg a day taken in several divided doses.

The safety and effectiveness of prazepam use in children under the age of eighteen has not been established.

Overdosage

Symptoms of a prazepam overdose may include coma, confusion, sleepiness, and slowed reflexes. If you experience any of these symptoms, go to the nearest hospital emergency room immediately.

Pregnancy and Lactation

Prazepam may cause birth defects. As a result, it should not be taken during pregnancy. If you are pregnant or plan to become pregnant, notify your doctor immediately.

The drug may pass into breast milk and may be harmful to a nursing infant. If the medication is essential to your health, your doctor may advise you not to breast-feed while you are taking it.

Protriptyline

Brand Name

Vivactil

General Information

Protriptyline is used in the treatment of depression. It is a member of the class of drugs called tricyclic antidepressants, which work by blocking the presynaptic reuptake of the neurotransmitters serotonin, norepinephrine, and dopamine in the brain. This suggests that many of the symptoms of depression may result from imbalances of one or more of these neurotransmitters.

Symptoms of depression include low, anxious, or "empty" feelings; loss of interest and pleasure in activities previously enjoyed; noticeable change of appetite; noticeable change in sleeping patterns; fatigue or loss of energy; feelings of hopelessness or pessimism; feelings of guilt, worthlessness, or helplessness; inability to concentrate, make decisions, or remember details; recurring thoughts of death or suicide, wishing to die or attempting suicide; and aches and pains, constipation, or other physical ailments that cannot be explained.

Side Effects

Side effects may include abdominal cramps; agitation; altered liver function; anorexia; anxiety; black tongue; blood disorders; blurred vision; breast development in males; breast enlargement and flow of milk in females; confusion; constipation; defective muscular coordination; delayed urination; delusions; diarrhea; dilated pupils; dilation of the urinary tract; disease of the nerves; disorientation; dizziness; drowsiness; drug fever; dry mouth; elevation or depression of blood sugar levels; fatigue; flushing; frequent urination; hair loss; headache; high blood pressure; high fever; impotence; incoordination; increased or decreased sex drive; increased pressure in the eyes; inflammation of the stomach; insomnia; irregular heartbeat; itching; low blood pressure; mild mania; nausea; nightmares; numbness or tingling of the extremities; palpitations; panic; paralysis of the intestines; peculiar taste; perspiration; purplish spots on the skin; rapid heartbeat; rash; restlessness; ringing in the ears; seizures; sensitivity to light; stroke; swelling due to fluid retention; swelling of the testicles; tingling; tremors; urinary retention; vomiting; weakness; weight gain or loss; worsening of psychosis; and yellowing of the skin and whites of the eyes.

If you experience any of these side effects or reactions, notify your doctor as soon as possible.

Important Precautions

Do not take protriptyline if you have had a heart attack recently, if you are taking a type of antidepressant called a monoamine oxidase inhibitor (MAOI) or have taken one within the past two weeks, or if you have ever had an allergic reaction or hypersensitivity to protriptyline or a similar drug.

Use this medication with caution if you have a history of cardiovascular disorders, hyperthyroidism, increased pressure in the eyes, seizures, or urinary retention.

Protriptyline may make you feel dizzy and drowsy. Do not drive, operate machinery, or participate in any high-risk activities until you know exactly how the drug affects you.

Since protriptyline can make you sensitive to light, try to stay out of the sun as much as possible during your treatment.

Abruptly discontinuing protriptyline may result in headaches, nausea, and malaise. When ending treatment with this medication, follow your doctor's schedule for a gradual withdrawal.

If possible, discontinue the drug several days before elective surgery.

Food and Drug Interactions

If protriptyline is taken with certain other drugs, the effects of either drug could be increased, decreased, or changed. Before beginning treatment with protriptyline, tell your doctor if you are taking any other prescription or over-the-counter medications.

Protriptyline should not be combined with MAOIs. It is also important to check with your doctor before taking protriptyline with anticholinergic drugs such as Artane and Cogentin, antipsychotic drugs, thyroid medications, cimetidine (Tagamet), or epinephrine (Epipen).

Protriptyline should not be taken with alcohol, sleeping pills, tranquilizers, or narcotic painkillers.

Recommended Dosage

Usual dosage for adults: The usual starting dose is 15 to 40 mg a day taken in three or four divided doses. If necessary, this amount may gradually be increased to 60 mg a day. Dosages above 60 mg are not recommended.

Usual dosage for adolescents and the elderly: The usual starting dose is 5 mg three times a day. If necessary, this amount may gradually be increased. In elderly people, the cardiovascular system must be monitored closely if the total daily dose exceeds 20 mg.

The safety and effectiveness of protriptyline use in children has not been established.

Overdosage

An overdose of protriptyline can be fatal. Symptoms of overdose may include agitation, below normal body temperature, coma, congestive heart failure, convulsions, dilated pupils, drowsiness, extremely low blood pressure, high fever, increased reflexes, muscle rigidity, rapid heartbeat, stupor, and vomiting. If you experience any of these symptoms, go to the nearest hospital emergency room immediately.

Pregnancy and Lactation

Protriptyline should only be used during pregnancy if the potential benefits clearly outweigh any potential risks to the fetus. If you are pregnant or plan to become pregnant, notify your doctor immediately.

The drug may pass into breast milk and may be harmful to a nursing infant. If the medication is essential to your health, your doctor may advise you not to breast-feed while you are taking it.

Quazepam

Brand Name
Doral

General Information

Quazepam is a sleeping pill prescribed for the short-term treatment of insomnia. It is a member of the class of drugs called benzodiazepines, which facilitate the action of the neurotransmitter GABA (gamma-aminobutyric acid). This leads to sedation, sleep, and relaxation of the large skeletal muscles.

Insomnia may involve difficulty falling asleep, waking up frequently during the night, and waking up early and not being able to get back to sleep.

Side Effects

Some people who have taken quazepam every night for several weeks suffer from increased wakefulness in the last third of the night and anxiety the next day.

On rare occasions, quazepam causes agitation, hallucinations, sleep disturbances, or stimulation. These symptoms indicate that you should discontinue therapy immediately.

More common side effects may include dizziness, drowsiness, dry mouth, fatigue, headache, and indigestion.

Less common side effects may include abdominal pain, abnormal taste, abnormal thinking, changes in sex drive, confusion, constipation, diarrhea, impotence, incontinence, irregular menstrual periods, irritability, itching, jaundice, muscle spasms, nervousness, nightmares, rash, slurred speech, urinary retention, vague feeling of being sick, vision problems, and weakness.

If you experience any of these side effects or reactions, notify your doctor as soon as possible.

Important Precautions

Do not take quazepam if you have ever had an allergic reaction or hypersensitivity to it or a similar drug, or if you know or think that you suffer from sleep apnea, a condition characterized by brief episodes of breathing cessation during sleep.

Use this medication with caution if you are severely depressed or if you have a history of alcohol or drug abuse.

The dose of quazepam that you take at night may make you less alert the next day. Do not drive, operate machinery, or participate in any high-risk activities until you know exactly how the drug affects you.

Quazepam is potentially addictive, even when used for a relatively short time. Consequently, you may experience withdrawal symptoms when you stop taking it. To help prevent withdrawal symptoms, do not abruptly discontinue quazepam. Instead, follow your doctor's schedule for a gradual tapering of the dosage.

Food and Drug Interactions

If quazepam is taken with certain other drugs, the effects of either drug could be increased, decreased, or changed. Before beginning treatment with quazepam, tell your doctor if you are taking any other prescription or over-the-counter medications.

It is particularly important to avoid combining

quazepam with any other medications that might slow the functioning of the central nervous system, including anticonvulsants, antihistamines, and antipsychotics.

Do not drink alcohol while taking quazepam.

Recommended Dosage

Usual dosage for adults: The usual starting dose is 15 mg at bedtime. This amount may later be decreased to 7.5 mg.

Dosages for the elderly should be determined by a doctor.

The safety and effectiveness of quazepam in children under the age of eighteen has not been established.

Overdosage

Symptoms of a quazepam overdose may include coma, confusion, and prolonged drowsiness. If you experience any of these symptoms, go to the nearest hospital emergency room immediately.

Pregnancy and Lactation

Quazepam may cause birth defects and/or withdrawal symptoms in infants. As a result, it should not be taken during pregnancy. If you are pregnant or plan to become pregnant, notify your doctor immediately.

The drug passes into breast milk and may be harmful to a nursing infant. As a result, it should not be taken while breast-feeding.

Risperidone

Brand Name

Risperdal

General Information

Risperidone is used in the treatment of psychotic disorders such as schizophrenia. It works by blocking the neurotransmitters dopamine and serotonin. This suggests that some of the symptoms of psychosis may result from abnormal dopamine and serotonin activity in the brain.

Symptoms of schizophrenia include delusions, hallucinations, disorganized speech, grossly disorganized or catatonic behavior, and absence of normal moods and emotions.

Side Effects

Risperidone may cause neuroleptic malignant syndrome (NMS), a rare but potentially life-threatening side effect characterized by severe muscle rigidity throughout the body. Other features of NMS include high fever, rapid heartbeat, rapid breathing, excessive perspiration, abnormal blood pressure, and kidney failure.

This drug also may cause a serious and at times permanent side effect called tardive dyskinesia. This neurological syndrome results in involuntary movements of the mouth, lips, and tongue such as tongue rolling, lip licking and smacking, chewing or sucking motions, pouting, and grimacing.

More common side effects may include abnormal

gait; anorexia; anxiety; constipation; decreased sex drive; diarrhea; dizziness; dry vagina; ejaculatory dysfunction; erectile dysfunction; excessive menstrual bleeding; excessive thirst; fatigue; increased dream activity; increased duration of sleep; increased muscular movement and physical activity; increased pigmentation; muscular weakness and rigidity; nausea; nervousness; painful digestion; rapid heartbeat; rash; reduced salivation; rhinitis; sensation of internal restlessness; sensitivity to light; severe and painful spasms of the muscles in the head and neck; sleepiness; urinary disturbances; and weight gain.

Less common side effects may include absence of menstruation; acne; amnesia; anemia; apathy; black stool; bleeding between menstrual periods; blood in the urine; breast enlargement; breast pain; catatonic reaction; confusion; coughing and wheezing; depression; diabetes mellitus; difficult and defective speech; euphoria; excessive gas in the stomach and intestines; flulike symptoms; hair loss; hemorrhoids; high blood pressure; hyperventilation; impaired concentration; inability to ejaculate; inability to swallow or difficulty in swallowing; increased appetite; increased or decreased sweating; increased sex drive; inflammation of the mouth or stomach; low blood pressure; malaise; nosebleed; overgrowth of the cornea; painful menstruation; painful or difficult urination; palpitations; perineal pain; pneumonia; severe itching; skin discoloration; spontaneous flow of milk; stupor; sudden chill and high temperature followed by sense of heat and profuse perspiration; swelling due to fluid retention; tenderness or pain in the muscles; thirst; unusually white or yellow mucous discharge from the cervical canal or vagina; urinary incontinence; vaginal bleeding; vertigo; and weight loss.

Rare side effects may include abnormal amount of phosphorous or uric acid in the blood; abnormal decrease of white blood cells; abnormal secretion and discharge of tears; abnormal sensitivity to sound; aggravated psoriasis; arthritis; asthma; bitter taste in mouth; bleeding from the gastrointestinal tract; boils; bone pain; breast development in males; bursitis; chest pain; coma; decreased hearing; decreased iron or decreased protein in the blood; dehydration; delirium; disease of the lymph nodes; discolored feces; diverticulitis; double vision; emotional swings; enlarged abdomen; excessive hair growth; extreme potassium depletion; eye pain; fecal incontinence; flushing; gallstones; heartburn; hepatitis; impairment of the ability to communicate through speech, writing, or signs; increased reflexes; increased sputum; increased triglycerides; inflammation of the bladder, the edges of the eyelids, the esophagus, the gallbladder, the gums, the skin, or the stomach and intestinal tract; jerky involuntary movements; joint disease; leg cramps; liver damage; liver failure; low blood sugar; male breast pain; migraine; nightmares; paleness; rapid heartbeat; rash; reduced kidney function; ringing in the ears; sensation of sparks or flashes of light; sensitivity to light; severe genital itching; skin ulceration; swelling of the tongue; tilting of the head to one side; tongue discoloration; tongue paralysis; tumor of the skin; urinary retention; vomiting of blood; withdrawal syndrome; and yawning.

If you experience any of these side effects or reactions, notify your doctor as soon as possible.

Important Precautions

Keep in mind that risperidone may cause neuroleptic malignant syndrome and tardive dyskinesia. It may also cause priapism, a potentially dangerous condition characterized by prolonged, painful erections.

Do not take risperidone if you have ever had an allergic reaction or hypersensitivity to it or a similar drug.

Use this medication with caution if you have a history of seizures, low blood pressure, or cardiovascular, kidney, or liver disease. Risperidone should also be used cautiously by people who are exposed to extreme heat.

Risperidone can mask the symptoms of brain tumors, intestinal blockage, and Reye's syndrome. Because it prevents vomiting, it can also mask the signs of an overdose of another drug.

This drug may make you feel drowsy and impair your coordination. Do not drive, operate machinery, or participate in any high-risk activities until you know exactly how it affects you.

Food and Drug Interactions

If risperidone is taken with certain other drugs, the effects of either drug could be increased, decreased, or changed. Before beginning treatment with risperidone, tell your doctor if you are taking any other prescription or over-the-counter medications.

It is particularly important to check with your doctor before taking risperidone with carbamazepine (Atretol, Tegretol), clozapine (Clozaril), antihypertensive medications, and drugs that act on the central nervous system.

Risperidone should not be combined with alcohol.

Recommended Dosage

Usual dosage for adults: The usual starting dose is 1 mg twice a day, followed by 1-mg increases on the second and third day, working up to a target dose of 3 mg twice a day. Once symptoms are under control, it should gradually be lowered to the minimum effective dose.

Usual dosage for the elderly: The usual starting dose is .5 mg twice a day since elderly people have a higher risk of developing tardive dyskinesia and low blood pressure. If necessary, this amount may be increased by increments of .5 mg twice a day.

The safety and effectiveness of risperidone use in children has not been established.

Overdosage

Symptoms of a risperidone overdose may include convulsions, extreme drowsiness, extremely low blood pressure, and rapid heartbeat. If you experience any of these symptoms, go to the nearest hospital emergency room immediately.

Pregnancy and Lactation

Risperidone should only be used during pregnancy if the potential benefits clearly outweigh any potential risks to the fetus. If you are pregnant or plan to become pregnant, notify your doctor immediately.

The drug may pass into breast milk and may be

harmful to a nursing infant. If the medication is essential to your health, your doctor may advise you not to breast-feed while you are taking it.

Sertraline

Brand Name
Zoloft

General Information
Sertraline is used to treat depression. It is also prescribed for the treatment of a wide variety of other conditions including attention deficit disorder, bulimia, obsessive-compulsive disorder, panic disorder, and phobias. However, it has not been approved by the FDA for these purposes.

It is a member of the class of drugs called selective serotonin reuptake inhibitors, which work by blocking the presynaptic reuptake of the neurotransmitter serotonin. This suggests that many of the symptoms of depression may result from abnormal serotonin activity in the brain.

Symptoms of depression include low, anxious, or "empty" feelings; loss of interest and pleasure in activities previously enjoyed; noticeable change of appetite; noticeable change in sleeping patterns; fatigue or loss of energy; feelings of hopelessness or pessimism; feelings of guilt, worthlessness, or helplessness; inability to concentrate, make decisions, or remember details; recurring thoughts of death or suicide, wishing to die or attempting suicide; and aches and pains, constipation, or other physical ailments that cannot be explained.

Side Effects

More common side effects may include confusion, diarrhea, or loose stools, difficulty with ejaculation, dizziness, dry mouth, fatigue, headache, increased perspiration, indigestion, insomnia, nausea, sleepiness, and tremors.

Less common side effects may include abdominal pain; abnormal hair growth; abnormal skin odor; acne; agitation; altered taste; anemia; anxiety; apathy; back pain; bad breath; belching; black stools; breast development in males; bruiselike marks on the skin; chest pain; clumsiness; cold, clammy skin; conjunctivitis; constipation; coughing; difficulty breathing, concentrating, swallowing, or walking; dilated pupils; double vision; dry eyes; dry skin; earache; enlarged abdomen; eye pain; fainting; feeling faint upon rising from a seated or prone position; fever; fluid retention; flushing; frequent urination; gas; hair loss; heart attack; hemorrhoids; hernia; hiccups; high or low blood pressure; hot flushes; increased appetite; increased salivation; inflammation of the nose, throat, tongue, or mouth; itching; joint pains; lack of coordination; lack of sensation; lethargy; loss of appetite; menstrual problems; middle-ear infection; migraine; muscle cramps or weakness; muscle pain; need to urinate during the night; nervousness; pain upon urination; pounding in the chest; racing heartbeat; rash; ringing in the ears; sensitivity to light, skin eruptions or inflammation; sores on the tongue; speech problems; stomach and intestinal inflammation; swelling around the eyes; swollen wrists and ankles; thirst; tingling sensation; twitching; urinary incontinence; vertigo; vomiting; weakness; weight gain or loss; and yawning.

Sertraline also may cause mental or emotional side effects including abnormal dreams or thoughts, aggressiveness, apathy, delusions, depersonalization (a feeling of "unreality"), euphoria, hallucinations, memory loss, paranoia, rapid mood swings, suicidal thoughts or attempted suicide, teeth grinding, and worsened depression.

If you experience any of these side effects or reactions, notify your doctor as soon as possible.

Important Precautions

Do not take sertraline if you are taking another type of antidepressant called a monoamine oxidase inhibitor (MAOI) or have taken one within the past two weeks, or if you have ever had an allergic reaction or hypersensitivity to sertraline or a similar drug.

Use this medication with caution if you have a history of seizures or kidney or liver disease.

Food and Drug Interactions

If sertraline is taken with certain other drugs, the effects of either drug could be increased, decreased, or changed. Before beginning treatment with sertraline, tell your doctor if you are taking any other prescription or over-the-counter medications.

Sertraline should not be combined with MAOIs. It is also important to check with your doctor before combining sertraline with over-the-counter medications, other psychiatric drugs, diazepam (Valium), lithium (Eskalith, Lithobid), tolbutamide (Orinase), or warfarin (Coumadin).

Do not drink alcohol while taking sertraline.

Recommended Dosage

Usual dosage for adults: The usual starting dose is 50 mg a day taken either in the morning or at night. This amount may be increased after several weeks if no improvement is noticed. Dosages above 200 mg a day are not recommended.

The safety and effectiveness of sertraline use in children has not been established.

Overdosage

Symptoms of overdose may include anxiety, dilated pupils, drowsiness, nausea, rapid heartbeat, and vomiting. If you experience any of these symptoms, go to the nearest hospital emergency room immediately.

Pregnancy and Lactation

The safety of sertraline use during pregnancy has not been established. As a result, it should only be taken during pregnancy if the potential benefits clearly outweigh any potential risks to the fetus. If you are pregnant or plan to become pregnant, notify your doctor immediately.

Studies have also not determined the safety of using sertraline during lactation. Consequently, the drug should only be used by a nursing mother if the potential benefits of therapy clearly outweigh any potential risks to the infant.

Tacrine

Brand Name
Cognex

General Information
Tacrine is used to treat dementia of the Alzheimer's-disease type. It works by increasing the availability of the neurotransmitter acetylcholine in the brain. This suggests that some of the symptoms of Alzheimer's disease may result from a deficiency of acetylcholine.

It is important to note, however, that tacrine has been demonstrated to be effective only for some patients, and even then, improvements in memory and other cognitive symptoms are usually only minimal. It must also be stressed that tacrine does not *cure* Alzheimer's disease, which has a progressive downhill course.

Side Effects
More common side effects may include abdominal pain; abnormal tension of the arteries or muscles; abnormal thinking; agitation; anorexia; anxiety; arthritis; back pain; bronchitis; chest pain; chills; confusion; conjunctivitis; constipation; convulsions; coughing; defective muscular coordination; depression; diarrhea; difficulty breathing; dizziness; excessive gas; fatigue; fever; flushing; hallucinations; headache; high blood pressure; hostility; incontinence; increased muscular movement and physical activity; increased

sweating; inflammation of the sinuses; insomnia; joint pain; lack or loss of strength; low blood pressure; malaise; nausea; nervousness; painful digestion; pneumonia; prolonged drowsiness; rash; rhinitis; sensation of numbness or tingling; skin discoloration; sudden breaking of a bone; swelling of the extremities; temporary loss of consciousness; tenderness or pain in the muscles; tremor; upper respiratory infection; urinary frequency; urinary tract infection; vertigo; vomiting; and weight loss.

Less common side effects may include abnormal dreams; abnormal gait; acne; amnesia; anemia; apathy; asthma; blood in the urine; bloody stools; boils; breast pain; bursitis; cataracts; chest congestion; chest pain; cyst; deafness; decreased or absent reflexes; dehydration; delirium; diabetes; difficult and defective speech; disease of the lymph nodes; disease of the nerves; diverticulitis; double vision; dry eyes; dry mouth or throat; dry skin; earache; eczema; excessive secretion and discharge of urine; excessive urination during the night; extreme slowness of movement; eye pain; facial swelling; fatty tumor; fecal impaction; fecal incontinence; gallstones; gastrointestinal bleeding; generalized swelling due to fluid retention; glaucoma; gout; hair loss; heart failure; hemorrhoids; herpes simplex; hiatal hernia; high cholesterol; hyperventilation; impairment of ability to communicate through speech, writing, or signs; impotence; inability to swallow or difficulty in swallowing; increased appetite, salivation, sensitivity to sensory stimuli, or increased sex drive; inflammation of a nerve, tendon, or vein; inflammation of the bladder, esophagus, gallbladder, gums, middle ear, mouth, skin, stomach, stomach and intestinal tract, or tongue; inner-ear infection; irregular heartbeat; kidney infection; kidney stones; lower respiratory infection; migraine; movement disorder; muscle weakness and rigidity; neurosis; nosebleed; osteoporosis; overgrowth of the cornea; painful or difficult urination; palpitations; paralysis of one side of the body; paranoia; prostate cancer; psoriasis; pus in the urine; rapid heartbeat; rectal bleeding; reduction or dimness of vision; ringing in the ears; severe genital itching; shingles; skin cancer; slow heartbeat; stomach ulcer; stroke; sugar in the urine; temporary interference with blood supply to the brain; twitching; unusual taste; urinary retention or urgency; vaginal bleeding; visual-field defect; wandering; and weight gain.

Rare side effects may include abnormal decrease of white blood cells; abnormal sensations on the skin; bladder tumor; bowel obstruction; breast cancer; cardiac arrest; coma; coughing up blood; dandruff; death; disease of skeletal muscles; duodenal ulcer; facial paralysis; heat exhaustion; hyperthyroidism; hypothyroidism; hysteria; inability to perform purposive movements; inability to sit still; inflammation of the brain, eyelids, or epididymis; inner-ear disturbance; involuntary fixation of the eyeballs; kidney failure; kidney tumor; loss of vision; lung cancer; lung swelling; malignant mole or tumor of the skin; ovarian cancer; prolonged muscle contractions; psychosis; shedding of the skin; skin necrosis; skin ulcer; slow, rhythmic movements; squamous-cell carcinoma; suicidal tendencies; and urinary obstruction.

If you experience any of these side effects or reactions, notify your doctor as soon as possible.

Important Precautions

Do not take tacrine if you have ever had an allergic reaction or hypersensitivity to it or a similar drug.

Use this medication with caution if you have a history of cardiovascular disease or liver dysfunction.

Because tacrine can cause liver damage, transaminase levels should be monitored once a week for at least the first eighteen weeks of treatment. After that time, monitoring may be reduced to once every three months. Whenever the dose of tacrine is increased, however, weekly monitoring should resume for a minimum of six weeks.

Abruptly discontinuing tacrine or dramatically reducing the total daily dose may lead to a decline in cognitive function and behavioral disturbances. As a result, dosage changes should not be made without instruction from a physician.

Food and Drug Interactions

If tacrine is taken with certain other drugs, the effects of either drug could be increased, decreased, or changed. Before beginning treatment with tacrine, tell your doctor if you are taking any other prescription or over-the-counter medications.

It is particularly important to check with your doctor before combining tacrine with cimetidine (Tagamet), theophylline (Theo-Dur), or anticholinergic drugs such as Artane and Cogentin.

Recommended Dosage

Usual dosage for adults: The usual starting dose is 40 mg a day. This dose should be maintained for a minimum of six weeks with weekly monitoring of transaminase levels. The dose should then be increased to 80 mg a day if there are no significant transaminase elevations and the patient is tolerating treatment. The dose should be increased to higher levels (120 and 160 mg a day) at six-week intervals based on tolerance.

Overdosage

Symptoms of a tacrine overdose may include collapse, convulsions, low blood pressure, muscle weakness, salivation, severe nausea and vomiting, slow heartbeat, and sweating. If you experience any of these symptoms, go to the nearest hospital emergency room immediately.

Pregnancy and Lactation

The safety of tacrine use during pregnancy has not been established. If you are pregnant or plan to become pregnant, notify your doctor immediately.

Tacrine may pass into breast milk and may be harmful to a nursing infant. If the medication is essential to your health, your doctor may advise you not to breast-feed while you are taking it.

Temazepam

Brand Name
Restoril

General Information
Temazepam is a sleeping pill prescribed for the short-term treatment of insomnia. It is a member of the class of drugs called benzodiazepines, which facilitate the action of the neurotransmitter GABA (gamma-aminobutyric acid). This leads to sedation, sleep, and relaxation of the large skeletal muscles.

Insomnia may involve difficulty falling asleep, waking up frequently during the night, or waking up early and not being able to get back to sleep.

Side Effects
More common side effects may include confusion, dizziness, drowsiness, exaggerated feeling of well-being, relaxed feeling, and sluggishness or unresponsiveness.

Less common or rare side effects may include diarrhea, excitement, falling, hallucinations, hyperactivity, involuntary eye movement, lack of concentration, lack of coordination, loss of appetite, loss of balance, rapid heartbeat, tremors, and weakness.

If you experience any of these side effects or reactions, notify your doctor as soon as possible.

Important Precautions

Do not take temazepam if you have ever had an allergic reaction or hypersensitivity to it or a similar drug.

Use this medication with caution if you are severely depressed or have a history of severe depression, if you have decreased kidney or liver function, or if you have chronic respiratory or lung disease. If you suffer from any of these conditions, be sure to discuss the details thoroughly with your doctor before taking temazepam.

The dose of temazepam that you take at night may make you drowsy and less alert the next day. Do not drive, operate machinery, or participate in any high-risk activities until you know exactly how the drug affects you.

Temazepam is potentially addictive even when used for a relatively short time. Consequently, you may experience withdrawal symptoms when you stop taking it. Withdrawal symptoms may include abdominal and muscle cramps, convulsions, feeling of discomfort, insomnia, sweating, tremors, and vomiting. To help prevent withdrawal symptoms, do not abruptly discontinue temazepam. Instead, follow your doctor's schedule for a gradual tapering of the dosage.

Food and Drug Interactions

If temazepam is taken with certain other drugs, the effects of either drug could be increased, decreased, or changed. Before beginning treatment with temazepam, tell your doctor if you are taking any other prescription or over-the-counter medications.

It is particularly important to avoid combining temazepam with any other medications that might slow the functioning of the central nervous system, including antihistamines and antianxiety agents.

Do not drink alcohol while taking temazepam.

Recommended Dosage

Usual dosage for adults: 15 mg at bedtime. Some people may only require 7.5 mg; others may require 30 mg. The dosage should be tailored to the individual. Dosages above 30 mg are not recommended.

Usual dosage for the elderly: The dosage should be limited to the minimum effective amount. The usual starting dose is 7.5 mg at bedtime.

The safety and effectiveness of temazepam use in children under the age of eighteen has not been established.

Overdosage

Symptoms of a temazepam overdose may include coma, confusion, decreased reflexes, labored or difficult breathing, loss of coordination, low blood pressure, seizures, sleepiness, and slurred speech. If you experience any of these symptoms, go to the nearest hospital emergency room immediately.

Pregnancy and Lactation

Temazepam may cause birth defects. As a result, it should not be taken during pregnancy. If you are pregnant or plan to become pregnant, notify your doctor immediately.

The drug may pass into breast milk and may be

harmful to a nursing infant. If the medication is essential to your health, your doctor may advise you not to breast-feed while you are taking it.

Thioridazine

Brand Name
Mellaril

General Information

Thioridazine is used in the treatment of psychotic disorders such as schizophrenia. It works by blocking the neurotransmitter dopamine. This suggests that many of the symptoms of psychosis may result from abnormal dopamine activity in the brain.

Symptoms of schizophrenia include delusions, hallucinations, disorganized speech, grossly disorganized or catatonic behavior, and absence of normal moods and emotions.

Side Effects

Thioridazine may cause neuroleptic malignant syndrome (NMS), a rare but potentially life-threatening side effect characterized by severe muscle rigidity throughout the body. Other features of NMS include high fever, rapid heartbeat, rapid breathing, excessive perspiration, abnormal blood pressure, and kidney failure.

This drug also may cause a serious, and at times permanent, side effect called tardive dyskinesia. This neurological syndrome results in involuntary movements of the mouth, lips, and tongue such as tongue rolling, lip licking and smacking, chewing or sucking motions, pouting, and grimacing.

Other side effects may include abnormal lack of movement; abnormal muscle rigidity; abnormal secretion of milk; agitation; altered mental state; anemia; asthma; blurred vision; breast development in males; changes in sex drive; chewing movements; confusion; constipation; diarrhea; difficulty urinating; discolored eyes; drowsiness; dry mouth; excitement; eye spasms; eyeball rotation or state of fixed gaze; fever; fluid retention and swelling; headache; inability to ejaculate; intestinal blockage; involuntary movements; irregular blood pressure, pulse, and heartbeat; irregular or missed menstrual periods; jaw spasm; loss or increase of appetite; masklike facial expression and rigidity; muscle rigidity; narrow pupils; nasal congestion; nausea; overactivity; pain in the shoulder and neck; painful muscle spasms; paleness; protruding tongue; psychotic reactions; puckering of the mouth; puffing of the cheeks; rapid heartbeat; redness of the skin; restlessness; rigid arms, feet, head, and muscles; sensitivity to light; skin itching, pigmentation, and rash; sluggishness; strange dreams; sweating; swelling of breasts; swelling of the throat; swollen glands; tremors; vomiting; weight gain; and yellowing of the skin and whites of the eyes.

If you experience any of these side effects or reactions, notify your doctor as soon as possible.

Important Precautions

Keep in mind that thioridazine can cause neuroleptic malignant syndrome and tardive dyskinesia.

Do not take thioridazine if you are also taking central nervous system depressants or if you have heart disease along with extremely high or low blood pressure.

Use this medication with caution if you have a history of glaucoma or heart, liver, lung, kidney, or thyroid disease. Thioridazine should also be used cautiously by people who are exposed to extreme heat or pesticides.

Thioridazine may make you feel drowsy and impair your coordination. Do not drive, operate machinery, or participate in any high-risk activities until you know exactly how the drug affects you.

Food and Drug Interactions

If thioridazine is taken with certain other drugs, the effects of either drug could be increased, decreased, or changed. Before beginning treatment with thioridazine, tell your doctor if you are taking any other prescription or over-the-counter medications.

It is particularly important to check with your doctor before taking thioridazine with epinephrine, pindolol (Visken), or propranolol (Inderal).

Thioridazine should not be combined with alcohol, narcotics, sleeping pills, or tranquilizers.

Recommended Dosage

Usual dosage for adults: The usual starting dose ranges from 150 to 300 mg a day taken in three divided doses. If necessary, this amount may be increased to a maximum of 800 mg a day taken in two to four divided doses. Once symptoms are under control, it should gradually be lowered to the minimum effective dose. Dosages above 800 mg a day should never be taken since higher doses have been associated with a condition called retinitis pigmentosa, which can injure the retina and even cause blindness.

Usual dosage for the elderly: The usual starting dose is 25 mg three times a day since elderly people have a higher risk of developing tardive dyskinesia. Average daily dosages range from 20 to 200 mg taken in two to four divided doses.

Usual dosage for children aged two to twelve: The usual starting dose is .5 mg to 3 mg per kilogram of body weight per day. Thioridazine is not recommended for children under the age of two.

Overdosage

Symptoms of a thioridazine overdose may include agitation, coma, convulsions, dry mouth, extreme drowsiness, extremely low blood pressure, fever, intestinal obstruction, irregular heart rate, and restlessness. If you experience any of these symptoms, go to the nearest hospital emergency room immediately.

Pregnancy and Lactation

Thioridazine should only be used during pregnancy if the potential benefits clearly outweigh any potential risks to the fetus. If you are pregnant or plan to become pregnant, notify your doctor immediately.

The drug may pass into breast milk and may be harmful to a nursing infant. If the medication is

essential to your health, your doctor may advise you not to breast-feed while you are taking it.

Thiothixene

Brand Name
Navane

General Information
Thiothixene is used in the treatment of psychotic disorders such as schizophrenia. It works by blocking the neurotransmitter dopamine. This suggests that many of the symptoms of psychosis may result from abnormal dopamine activity in the brain.

Symptoms of schizophrenia include delusions, hallucinations, disorganized speech, grossly disorganized or catatonic behavior, and absence of normal moods and emotions.

Side Effects
Thiothixene may cause neuroleptic malignant syndrome (NMS), a rare but potentially life-threatening side effect characterized by severe muscle rigidity throughout the body. Other features of NMS include high fever, rapid heartbeat, rapid breathing, excessive perspiration, abnormal blood pressure, and kidney failure.

This drug may also cause a serious and at times permanent side effect called tardive dyskinesia. This neurological syndrome results in involuntary movements of the mouth, lips, and tongue such as tongue rolling, lip licking and smacking, chewing or sucking motions, pouting, and grimacing.

Other side effects may include abnormal muscle rigidity; abnormal secretion of milk; abnormalities of movement and posture; agitation; anemia; blurred vision; breast development in males; chewing movements; constipation; diarrhea; dizziness; drowsiness; dry mouth; excessive thirst; eyeball rotation or state of fixed gaze; fainting; fatigue; fever; fluid retention and swelling; headache; high or low blood sugar; hives, impotence; insomnia; intestinal blockage; irregular menstrual periods; itching; light-headedness; loss or increase of appetite; low blood pressure; narrow or dilated pupils; nasal congestion; nausea; painful muscle spasms; protruding tongue; puckering of the mouth; puffing of the cheeks; rapid heartbeat; rash; restlessness; salivation; sedation; seizures; sensitivity to light; skin inflammation and peeling; sweating; swelling of breasts; tremors; twitching in the body, neck, shoulders, and face; visual problems; vomiting; weakness; weight gain; and worsening of psychotic symptoms.

If you experience any of these side effects or reactions, notify your doctor as soon as possible.

Important Precautions

Keep in mind that thiothixene can cause neuroleptic malignant syndrome and tardive dyskinesia.

Do not take thiothixene if you have a known hypersensitivity to it, if your central nervous system is depressed, if you have suffered a circulatory-system collapse, or if you have a bone-marrow or blood disorder.

Thiothixene can mask the symptoms of brain tumors and intestinal blockages. Use this medication with caution if you have a history of brain tumors, breast cancer, convulsive disorders, glaucoma, heart disease, or intestinal obstruction. Thiothixene should also be used cautiously by people who are exposed to extreme heat or are recovering from alcoholism.

The drug may make you feel dizzy and drowsy. Do not drive, operate machinery, or participate in any high-risk activities until you know exactly how it affects you.

Food and Drug Interactions

If thiothixene is taken with certain other drugs, the effects of either drug could be increased, decreased, or changed. Before beginning treatment with thiothixene, tell your doctor if you are taking any other prescription or over-the-counter medications.

It is particularly important to check with your doctor before taking thiothixene with antihistamines or atropine (Donnatal).

Thiothixene should not be combined with alcohol, narcotics, sleeping pills, or tranquilizers.

Recommended Dosage

Usual dosage for adults: The usual starting dose is 6 mg a day taken in three divided doses for mild symptoms. If necessary, this amount may be increased to 15 mg a day. For more severe symptoms, the usual starting dose is 10 mg a day taken in two divided doses. If necessary, this amount may be increased to 60 mg a day.

Elderly people usually take lower doses of thiothixene since they have a higher risk of developing tardive dyskinesia and low blood pressure.

Thiothixene is not recommended for children under the age of twelve.

Overdosage

Symptoms of a thiothixene overdose may include coma, difficulty swallowing, headed tilted to the side, low blood pressure, muscle rigidity, salivation, tremors, walking problems, and weakness. If you experience any of these symptoms, go to the nearest hospital emergency room immediately.

Pregnancy and Lactation

Thiothixene should only be used during pregnancy if the potential benefits clearly outweigh any potential risks to the fetus. If you are pregnant or plan to become pregnant, notify your doctor immediately.

The drug may pass into breast milk and may be harmful to a nursing infant. If the medication is essential to your health, your doctor may advise you not to breast-feed while you are taking it.

Tranylcypromine

Brand Name
Parnate

General Information

Tranylcypromine is used to treat depression. It is a member of the class of drugs called monoamine oxidase inhibitors (MAOIs). Monoamine oxidase is an enzyme that breaks down the neurotransmitters serotonin, norepinephrine, and dopamine. Tranylcypromine helps to create more balanced moods by blocking the effects of monoamine oxidase. Unfortunately, blocking monoamine oxidase throughout the entire body can cause serious side effects if a patient is not scrupulously careful about avoiding certain foods and medications. For this reason, MAOIs are typically reserved for situations in which other antidepressant drug treatments have failed.

Symptoms of depression include low, anxious, or "empty" feelings; loss of interest and pleasure in activities previously enjoyed; noticeable change of appetite; noticeable change in sleeping patterns; fatigue or loss of energy; feelings of hopelessness or pessimism; feelings of guilt, worthlessness, or helplessness; inability to concentrate, make decisions, or remember details; recurring thoughts of death or suicide, wishing to die or attempting suicide; and aches and pains, constipation, or other physical ailments that cannot be explained.

Side Effects

Side effects may include abdominal pain; anorexia; blood disorders; blurred vision; chills; constipation; diarrhea; dizziness, drowsiness; dry mouth; headache; hepatitis; impotence; insomnia; low blood pressure; muscle spasms or twitches; nausea; numbness; palpitations; rapid heartbeat; rash; restlessness; retarded ejaculation; ringing in the ears; sensation of prickling or tingling; swelling due to fluid retention; tremors; urinary retention; and weakness.

If you experience any of these side effects or reactions, notify your doctor as soon as possible.

Important Precautions

Taking tranylcypromine with certain foods, beverages, and medications can cause serious, potentially fatal, high blood pressure. For detailed information on substances to avoid, see the "Food and Drug Interactions" section below.

Do not take tranylcypromine if you are taking another monoamine oxidase inhibitor or have taken one within the past week; if you have a confirmed or suspected cerebrovascular defect, cardiovascular disease, hypertension, liver disease, or pheochromocytoma (a small tumor of the adrenal gland); if you are over the age of sixty; or if you have ever had an allergic reaction or hypersensitivity to tranylcypromine or a similar drug.

Use this medication with caution if you have diabetes or hyperthyroidism.

Promptly report any unusual symptoms such as headache, palpitations and/or rapid heartbeat, a sense of constriction in the throat or chest, sweating, dizziness, stiff neck, nausea, or vomiting to your doctor. These symptoms may indicate that treatment with tranylcypromine should be discontinued.

Tranylcypromine may make you feel dizzy and drowsy. Do not drive, operate machinery, or participate in any high-risk activities until you know exactly how the drug affects you.

Be sure to inform your doctor or dentist that you are taking tranylcypromine, or have taken it within the past two weeks, before having any type of surgery or dental treatment. Do not undergo elective surgery requiring anesthesia while you are on the drug. Always carry a card or wear a bracelet that says you take tranylcypromine.

Food and Drug Interactions

If tranylcypromine is taken with certain other drugs, the effects of either drug could be increased, decreased, or changed. Before beginning treatment with tranylcypromine, tell your doctor if you are taking any other prescription or over-the-counter medications.

The use of any MAOI requires patients to observe rigid dietary restrictions since foods containing a naturally occurring substance called tyramine can interact with the drug and trigger a sudden, potentially life-threatening rise in blood pressure. Foods to avoid while taking tranylcypromine, and for one week after discontinuing treatment with the medication, include beer (including alcohol-free or reduced-alcohol brands); caffeine (in excessive amounts); cheese (except for cottage cheese and cream cheese); dry sausage (including salami and pepperoni); fava beans; liver; meat extract; pickled, fermented, aged, or smoked meat, fish, or dairy products; pickled herring; sauerkraut; wine (including alcohol-free and reduced-alcohol brands); yeast extract (including large amounts of brewer's yeast); and yogurt.

A number of prescription and over-the-counter drugs must be avoided as well, including amphetamines, appetite suppressants, asthma inhalants, central nervous system stimulants, cold and cough preparations, hay fever medications, nasal decongestants, other antidepressants, products containing L-tryptophan, sinus medications, and weight-loss preparations. For a complete list of prohibited foods, beverages, and medications, see your doctor.

Tranylcypromine should not be combined with alcohol, sleeping pills, tranquilizers, or narcotic pain-killers.

Recommended Dosage

Usual dosage for adults: The usual starting dose is 30 mg a day taken in divided doses. If necessary, this amount may gradually be increased to a maximum of 60 mg a day.

Dosages for children and the elderly should be individually tailored by a doctor.

Overdosage

Symptoms of a tranylcypromine overdose are usually the same as the side effects listed above. Some people, however, experience an intensification of these symptoms and/or additional symptoms such as agitation, extreme dizziness, incoherence, mental confusion, severe headache, and shock. If you experience any of these symptoms, go to the nearest hospital emergency room immediately.

Pregnancy and Lactation

The safety of tranylcypromine use during pregnancy has not been established. As a result, it should only be taken during pregnancy if the potential benefits clearly outweigh any potential risks to the fetus. If you are pregnant or plan to become pregnant, notify your doctor immediately.

The drug passes into breast milk and may be harmful to a nursing infant. If the medication is essential to your health, your doctor may advise you not to breast-feed while you are taking it.

Trazodone

Brand Name
Desyrel

General Information

Trazodone is used to treat depression with or without anxiety. While its mechanism of action is unknown, it is believed to work by facilitating the action of the neurotransmitter serotonin. This suggests that many of the symptoms of depression may result from abnormal serotonin activity in the brain.

Symptoms of depression include low, anxious, or "empty" feelings; loss of interest and pleasure in activities previously enjoyed; noticeable change of appetite; noticeable change in sleeping patterns; fatigue or loss of energy; feelings of hopelessness or pessimism; feelings of guilt, worthlessness, or helplessness; inability to concentrate, make decisions, or remember details; recurring thoughts of death or suicide, wishing to die or attempting suicide; and aches and pains, constipation, or other physical ailments that cannot be explained.

Side Effects

Trazodone has been linked to a condition called priapism, which is a prolonged, painful erection of the penis. Men who experience persistent or inappropriate erections should stop taking the drug and notify their doctor.

More common side effects may include abdominal or stomach disorders; aches or pains in muscles or bones; allergic skin reaction; anger or hostility; bad taste in the mouth; blurred vision; brief loss of consciousness; confusion; constipation; decreased appetite, concentration, or sex drive; diarrhea; disorientation; dizziness or light-headedness; drowsiness; dry mouth; excitement; fatigue; fluid retention and swelling; fullness or heaviness in the head; headache; high or low blood pressure; impaired memory; insomnia; nasal or sinus congestion; nausea or vomiting; nervousness; nightmares or vivid dreams; rapid heartbeat; red, tired, itchy eyes; shortness of breath; sudden loss of strength or fainting; sweating or clammy skin; tingling sensation; tremors; uncoordinated movements; and weight gain or loss.

Less common or rare side effects may include agitation; anemia; blood in the urine; breast enlargement; chest pain; delayed urine flow; double vision; early or missed menstrual periods; ejaculation abnormalities;

excess salivation; gas; grand mal seizures; hair loss; hallucinations or delusions; heart attack; impaired speech; impotence; increased appetite, sex drive, or urinary frequency; jaundice; lack of muscle coordination; liver disorders; mild degree of mania or elevated mood; milk production; muscle twitches; numbness; prolonged erections; rash and itching; restlessness; slow heartbeat; swelling due to fluid retention; temporary interruption of normal breathing; and weakness.

If you experience any of these side effects or reactions, notify your doctor as soon as possible.

Important Precautions

Keep in mind that trazodone can cause priapism.

Do not take trazodone if you have ever had an allergic reaction or hypersensitivity to it or a similar drug.

Trazodone may make you feel dizzy and drowsy. Do not drive, operate machinery, or participate in any high-risk activities until you know exactly how the drug affects you.

Be sure to inform your doctor or dentist that you are taking trazodone before having any type of surgery or dental treatment. Do not undergo elective surgery requiring anesthesia while you are on the drug.

Food and Drug Interactions

If trazodone is taken with certain other drugs, the effects of either drug could be increased, decreased, or changed. Before beginning treatment with trazodone, tell your doctor if you are taking any other prescription or over-the-counter medications.

It is particularly important to check with your

doctor before taking trazodone with digoxin (Lanoxin), phenytoin (Dilantin), barbiturates, high blood pressure medications, a type of antidepressant called a monoamine oxidase inhibitor, or any other antidepressants.

Do not drink alcohol while taking trazodone.

Recommended Dosage

Usual dosage for adults: The usual starting dose is a total of 150 mg a day taken in two or more doses. This amount may be increased by 50 mg every three or four days. Dosages above 400 mg a day are not recommended. Once the maximum therapeutic benefit has been reached, the dosage may gradually be lowered.

Dosages for the elderly should be determined by a doctor.

The safety and effectiveness of trazodone use in children has not been established.

Overdosage

An overdose of trazodone can be fatal when it is combined with other drugs. Symptoms of overdose may include breathing failure; drowsiness; irregular heartbeat; prolonged, painful erection; seizures; and vomiting. If you experience any of these symptoms, go to the nearest hospital emergency room immediately.

Pregnancy and Lactation

The safety of trazodone use during pregnancy has not been established. As a result, it should only be taken during pregnancy if the potential benefits clearly outweigh any potential risks to the fetus. If you are pregnant or plan to become pregnant, notify your doctor immediately.

The drug may pass into breast milk and may be harmful to a nursing infant. If the medication is essential to your health, your doctor may advise you not to breast-feed while you are taking it.

Triazolam

Brand Name

Halcion

General Information

Triazolam is a sleeping pill prescribed for the short-term treatment of insomnia. It is a member of the class of drugs called benzodiazepines, which facilitate the action of the neurotransmitter GABA (gamma-aminobutyric acid). This leads to sedation, sleep, and relaxation of the large skeletal muscles.

Insomnia may involve difficulty falling asleep, waking up frequently during the night, or waking up early and not being able to get back to sleep.

Side Effects

Some people experience increased anxiety during the daytime while taking triazolam.

If you suffer from unusual, disturbing thoughts or behavior during triazolam therapy, inform your doctor immediately.

More common side effects may include dizziness, drowsiness, headache, light-headedness, nausea, nervousness, and vomiting.

Less common or rare side effects may include aggressiveness; agitation; behavior problems; burning tongue; changes in sex drive; chest pain; confusion; congestion; constipation; cramps; delusions; depression including suicidal thoughts; diarrhea; disorientation; dream abnormalities; dry mouth; exaggerated feeling of well-being; excitement; fainting; falling; fatigue; hallucinations; impaired urination; inappropriate behavior; incontinence; inflammation of the tongue and mouth; irritability; itching; loss of appetite; loss of sense of reality; memory impairment; memory loss; menstrual irregularities; morning hangover effects; muscle spasms in the shoulders or neck; nightmares; rapid heart rate; restlessness; ringing in the ears; skin inflammation; sleep disturbances including insomnia or sleepwalking; slurred or difficult speech; stiff and awkward movements; taste changes; tingling sensation; tiredness; visual problems; weakness; and yellowing of the skin and whites of the eyes.

If you experience any of these side effects or reactions, notify your doctor as soon as possible.

Important Precautions

Do not take triazolam if you have ever had an allergic reaction or hypersensitivity to it or a similar drug.

Use this medication with caution if you have a history of alcoholism, drug abuse, or personality disorders; if you have kidney, liver, or lung problems; or if you suffer from sleep apnea, a condition characterized by brief episodes of breathing cessation during sleep.

The dose of triazolam that you take at night may make you drowsy and less alert the next day. Do not drive, operate machinery, or participate in any high-risk activities until you know exactly how the drug affects you.

"Traveler's amnesia" has been experienced by people who used triazolam to fall asleep while traveling on airplanes. To prevent this reaction, take triazolam only when it is possible for you to get a full night of sleep.

Triazolam is potentially addictive even when used for a relatively short time. Consequently, you may experience withdrawal symptoms when you stop taking it. Withdrawal symptoms may include convulsions, cramps, insomnia, perceptual problems, sweating, tremors, and vomiting. To help prevent withdrawal symptoms, do not abruptly discontinue triazolam. Instead, follow your doctor's schedule for a gradual tapering of the dosage.

After ending treatment with triazolam, you may experience "rebound insomnia," a bad case of insomnia that lingers until a normal sleep pattern is reestablished—usually a few nights.

Food and Drug Interactions

If triazolam is taken with certain other drugs, the effects of either drug could be increased, decreased, or changed. Before beginning treatment with triazolam, tell your doctor if you are taking any other prescription or over-the-counter medications.

Do not drink alcohol while taking triazolam. This combination could result in excessive drowsiness and other potentially hazardous side effects such as respiratory depression, which can be fatal.

For the same reason, it is important to avoid combining triazolam with any other medications that might slow the functioning of the central nervous system, including anticonvulsants, antihistamines, antipsychotics, and barbiturates. Taking triazolam with cimetidine (Tagamet), the antibiotic erythromycin, or monoamine oxidase inhibitors is also not recommended.

Recommended Dosage

Usual dosage for adults: .25 mg before bedtime. Dosages above .5 mg are not recommended.

Usual dosage for the elderly: The dosage should be limited to the minimum effective amount. The usual starting dose is .125 mg at bedtime. If necessary, it may be increased to .25 mg.

The safety and effectiveness of triazolam use in children under the age of eighteen has not been established.

Overdosage

A severe overdose of triazolam can be fatal. Symptoms of overdose may include coma, confusion, coordination problems, excessive sleepiness, seizures, shallow or difficult breathing, and slurred speech. If you experience any of these symptoms, go to the nearest hospital emergency room immediately.

Pregnancy and Lactation

Triazolam may cause birth defects. As a result, it should not be taken during pregnancy. If you are pregnant or plan to become pregnant, notify your doctor immediately.

The drug may pass into breast milk and may be harmful to a nursing infant. As a result, it should not be taken while breast-feeding.

Trifluoperazine

Brand Name
Stelazine

General Information

Trifluoperazine is used to treat psychotic disorders such as schizophrenia. It works by blocking the neurotransmitter dopamine. This suggests that many of the symptoms of psychosis may result from abnormal dopamine activity in the brain.

Symptoms of schizophrenia include delusions, hallucinations, disorganized speech, grossly disorganized or catatonic behavior, and absence of normal moods and emotions.

Side Effects

Trifluoperazine may cause neuroleptic malignant syndrome (NMS), a rare but potentially life-threatening side effect characterized by severe muscle rigidity throughout the body. Other features of NMS include high fever, rapid heartbeat, rapid breathing, excessive perspiration, abnormal blood pressure, and kidney failure.

This drug may also cause a serious and at times permanent side effect called tardive dyskinesia. This neurological syndrome results in involuntary movements of the mouth, lips, and tongue such as tongue rolling, lip licking and smacking, chewing or sucking motions, pouting, and grimacing.

Other side effects may include abnormal secretion of milk; abnormal sugar in urine; abnormalities of movement and posture; agitation; anemia; asthma; blood disorders; blurred vision; breast development in males; catatonic states; chewing movements; constipation; difficulty swallowing; dizziness; drowsiness; dry mouth; ejaculation problems; exaggerated reflexes; excessive or spontaneous flow of milk; eye problems causing a state of fixed gaze; eye spasms; fatigue; fever; flulike symptoms; fluid accumulation in the brain; fluid retention and swelling; fragmented movements; head bent backward; headache; heart attack; high or low blood sugar; hives; impotence;

increase in appetite; infections; insomnia; intestinal blockage; involuntary movements of arms and legs; irregular blood pressure, pulse, and heartbeat; irregular or absence of menstrual periods; light-headedness; loss of appetite; low blood pressure; masklike facial expression; muscle stiffness and rigidity; narrow or dilated pupils; nasal congestion; nausea; pain and stiffness in the neck; persistent, painful erections; protruding tongue; psychotic symptoms; puckering of the mouth; puffing of the cheeks; rapid heartbeat; red blood spots; restlessness; rigid arms, feet, head, and muscles; seizures; sensitivity to light; shock; shuffling gait; skin inflammation and peeling; skin itching, pigmentation, and rash; spasms in the jaw, face, tongue, back, and mouth; sweating; swelling of the throat; tremors; twisted neck; weakness; weight gain; and yellowing of the skin and whites of the eyes.

If you experience any of these side effects or reactions, notify your doctor as soon as possible.

Important Precautions

Keep in mind that trifluoperazine can cause neuroleptic malignant syndrome and tardive dyskinesia.

Do not take trifluoperazine if you are also taking central nervous system depressants, if you have liver damage, or if you have a bone-marrow or blood disorder.

Use this medication with caution if you have a history of brain tumors, breast cancer, glaucoma, heart or liver disease, intestinal obstruction, or seizures. Trifluoperazine should also be used cautiously by people who are exposed to extreme heat or pesticides.

If you develop a fever or sore throat, mouth, or gums while taking trifluoperazine, inform your doctor immediately. These symptoms may indicate that you need to discontinue therapy.

Trifluoperazine can mask the symptoms of brain tumors, intestinal blockage, and Reye's syndrome.

The drug may make you feel dizzy and drowsy. Do not drive, operate machinery, or participate in any high-risk activities until you know exactly how it affects you.

Some people develop an allergic reaction to a sulfite contained in trifluoperazine.

Abruptly discontinuing trifluoperazine may result in dizziness, loss of appetite, nausea, tremors, and vomiting. When ending treatment with this medication, follow your doctor's schedule for a gradual withdrawal.

Food and Drug Interactions

If trifluoperazine is taken with certain other drugs, the effects of either drug could be increased, decreased, or changed. Before beginning treatment with trifluoperazine, tell your doctor if you are taking any other prescription or over-the-counter medications.

It is particularly important to check with your doctor before taking trifluoperazine with anticoagulants, anticonvulsants, antihistamines, barbiturates, certain diuretics, atropine (Donnatal), guanethidine (Ismelin), and propranolol (Inderal).

Trifluoperazine should not be combined with alcohol, narcotics, sleeping pills, or tranquilizers.

Recommended Dosage

Usual dosage for adults: The usual starting dose is 4 to 10 mg a day taken in two divided doses. Average doses range from 15 to 40 mg a day.

Elderly people usually take lower doses of trifluoperazine since they have a higher risk of developing tardive dyskinesia and low blood pressure.

Usual dosage for children aged six to twelve: The usual starting dose is 1 mg once or twice a day. Dosages above 15 mg are generally not required.

Overdosage

Symptoms of a trifluoperazine overdose may include agitation, coma, convulsions, difficulty breathing, difficulty swallowing, dry mouth, extreme sleepiness, fever, intestinal obstruction, irregular heart rate, low blood pressure, and restlessness. If you experience any of these symptoms, go to the nearest hospital emergency room immediately.

Pregnancy and Lactation

The safety of trifluoperazine use during pregnancy has not been established. As a result, it should only be taken during pregnancy if the potential benefits clearly outweigh any potential risks to the fetus. If you are pregnant or plan to become pregnant, notify your doctor immediately.

The drug passes into breast milk and may be harmful to a nursing infant. If the medication is essential to your health, your doctor may advise you not to breast-feed while you are taking it.

Trimipramine

Brand Name
Surmontil

General Information
Trimipramine is used to treat depression. It is a member of the class of drugs called tricyclic antidepressants, which work by blocking the presynaptic reuptake of the neurotransmitters serotonin, norepinephrine, and dopamine in the brain. This suggests that many of the symptoms of depression may result from imbalances of one or more of these neurotransmitters.

Symptoms of depression include low, anxious, or "empty" feelings; loss of interest and pleasure in activities previously enjoyed; noticeable change of appetite; noticeable change in sleeping patterns; fatigue or loss of energy; feelings of hopelessness or pessimism; feelings of guilt, worthlessness, or helplessness; inability to concentrate, make decisions, or remember details; recurring thoughts of death or suicide, wishing to die or attempting suicide; and aches and pains, constipation, or other physical ailments that cannot be explained.

Side Effects
Side effects may include abdominal cramps; agitation; anxiety; black tongue; blood disorders; blurred vision; breast development in males; breast enlargement in females; confusion; constipation; delusions;

diarrhea; difficult or frequent urination; dilated pupils; disorientation; dizziness; drowsiness; dry mouth; excessive or spontaneous flow of milk; fatigue; fever; flushing; hair loss; hallucinations; headache; heart attack; high or low blood pressure; high or low blood sugar; hives; impotence; increased or decreased sex drive; increased psychotic symptoms; inflamed lymph gland under the tongue; inflammation of the mouth; insomnia; intestinal blockage; irregular or pounding heartbeat; itching; lack of coordination; loss of appetite; nausea; nightmares; numbness; odd taste in mouth; perspiration; purple or reddish brown spots on the skin; rash; restlessness; ringing in the ears; seizures; sensitivity to light; sore throat; stomach upset; stroke; swelling of the face and tongue; swelling of the testicles; swollen glands; tingling sensation; tremors; visual problems; vomiting; weakness; weight gain or loss; and yellowing of the skin and whites of the eyes.

If you experience any of these side effects or reactions, notify your doctor as soon as possible.

Important Precautions

Do not take trimipramine if you have had a heart attack recently, if you are taking another type of antidepressant called a monoamine oxidase inhibitor (MAOI) or have taken one within the past two weeks, or if you have ever had an allergic reaction or hypersensitivity to trimipramine or a similar drug.

Use this medication with caution if you have a history of heart, liver, or thyroid disease, seizures, glaucoma, or urinary retention.

Trimipramine may make you feel dizzy and drowsy. Do not drive, operate machinery, or participate in any high-risk activities until you know exactly how the drug affects you.

Abruptly discontinuing trimipramine may result in headaches, nausea, and other unpleasant side effects. When ending treatment with this medication, follow your doctor's schedule for a gradual withdrawal.

Food and Drug Interactions

If trimipramine is taken with certain other drugs, the effects of either drug could be increased, decreased, or changed. Before beginning treatment with trimipramine, tell your doctor if you are taking any other prescription or over-the-counter medications.

Trimipramine should not be combined with MAOIs. It is also important to check with your doctor before combining trimipramine with anticholinergic drugs such as Artane and Cogentin, catecholamines (epinephrine and norepinephrine), local anesthetics, local decongestants, oral nasal decongestants, thyroid medications, cimetidine (Tagamet), and guanethidine (Ismelin).

Trimipramine should not be taken with alcohol.

Recommended Dosage

Usual starting dosage for adults: 75 mg a day taken in divided doses. If necessary, this amount may gradually be increased to 150 mg a day divided into equal smaller doses. Dosages above 200 mg a day are not recommended.

Usual maintenance dosage for adults: 50 to 150 mg a day taken in one dose at bedtime or several divided doses throughout the day.

Usual dosage for adolescents and the elderly: The

usual starting dose is 50 mg a day. If necessary, this amount may be increased to 100 mg a day.

Trimipramine is not recommended for children.

Overdosage

An overdose of trimipramine can be fatal. Symptoms of overdose may include agitation, bluish skin, breathing difficulty, coma, convulsions, dilated pupils, drowsiness, fever, heart failure, involuntary movement, irregular heart rate, lack of coordination, low blood pressure, rapid heartbeat, restlessness, rigid muscles, shock, stupor, sweating, and vomiting. If you experience any of these symptoms, go to the nearest hospital emergency room immediately.

Pregnancy and Lactation

Trimipramine should only be used during pregnancy if the potential benefits clearly outweigh any potential risks to the fetus. If you are pregnant or plan to become pregnant, notify your doctor immediately.

The drug also may pass into breast milk and may be harmful to a nursing infant. If the medication is essential to your health, your doctor may advise you not to breast-feed while you are taking it.

Valproic Acid

Brand Names
Depakene, Depakote

General Information
Valproic acid is an anticonvulsant drug used in the treatment of seizure disorders such as epilepsy. Depakote was also recently approved for treatment of the manic episodes associated with bipolar disorder. Valproic acid may work via effects on the neurotransmitter GABA (gamma-aminobutyric acid).

Symptoms of mania include elation, hyperactivity, flight of ideas, rapid speech, grandiose ideas, hostility, decreased need for sleep, and uncharacteristically poor judgment.

Side Effects
Common side effects of valproic acid may include indigestion, nausea, and vomiting. Depakote in particular may also cause a change in menstrual periods, drowsiness, temporary hair loss, and weight gain.

Less common or rare side effects of valproic acid may include abdominal cramps; anemia; behavior changes; bleeding; blood disorders; bruising; constipation; depression; diarrhea; dizziness; double vision; emotional upset; fluid retention; headache; involuntary eye movements; itching; lack of muscular coordination; liver disease; loss of appetite; sensitivity to light; skin rash; speech difficulties; spots before the eyes; tremors; and weakness.

If you experience any of these side effects or reactions, notify your doctor as soon as possible.

Important Precautions

Valproic acid can cause liver failure. As a result, liver-function tests must be performed before you begin taking the drug and throughout treatment. Symptoms of liver failure include facial swelling, lethargy, loss of appetite, vomiting, and weakness.

Since valproic acid can also lead to blood disorders, your blood must be monitored regularly while you are taking the drug. Bruising, clotting, or hemorrhaging usually means the dosage should be decreased or the medication should be discontinued.

Do not take valproic acid if you have a history of liver disease or liver dysfunction or if you have ever had an allergic reaction to this drug or a similar drug.

This medication makes some people feel dizzy and drowsy. Do not drive, operate machinery, or participate in any high-risk activities until you know exactly how the drug affects you.

Be sure to inform your doctor or dentist that you are taking valproic acid before undergoing any type of surgery or dental treatment.

To avoid stomach upset, take valproic acid with food.

Food and Drug Interactions

If valproic acid is taken with certain other drugs, the effects of either drug could be increased, decreased, or changed. Before beginning treatment with valproic acid, tell your doctor if you are taking any other prescription or over-the-counter medications.

It is particularly important to check with your

doctor before combining valproic acid with aspirin, blood thinners, oral contraceptives, or other anticonvulsant medications such as carbamazepine (Tegretol), clonazepam (Klonopin), ethosuximide (Zarontin), phenobarbital (Donnatal), phenytoin (Dilantin), and primidone (Mysoline).

Valproic acid should not be taken with alcohol or sleeping pills.

Recommended Dosage

The recommended daily dose of valproic acid depends upon the condition that is being treated. A blood test will help your doctor determine the proper dosage. It is generally built up slowly to minimize gastric upset.

Usual dosage: 15 to 60 mg per 2.2 pounds of body weight.

Overdosage

The primary symptom of a valproic acid overdose is a deep coma. If you suspect that you've taken too much of the drug, go to the nearest hospital emergency room immediately.

Pregnancy and Lactation

Valproic acid can cause birth defects. For this reason, it should only be used during pregnancy if the potential benefit clearly outweighs the potential risk. If you are pregnant or plan to become pregnant, notify your doctor immediately.

The drug also passes into breast milk and may be harmful to a nursing infant. If the medication is

essential to your health, your doctor may advise you not to breast-feed while you are taking it.

Venlafaxine

Brand Name
Effexor

General Information
Venlafaxine, which is used to treat depression, is chemically unrelated to any other antidepressants on the market. It works by blocking the presynaptic reuptake of the neurotransmitters serotonin and norepinephrine in the brain. This suggests that many of the symptoms of depression may result from abnormalities in both serotonin and norepinephrine activity in the brain.

Symptoms of depression include low, anxious, or "empty" feelings; loss of interest and pleasure in activities previously enjoyed; noticeable change of appetite; noticeable change in sleeping patterns; fatigue or loss of energy; feelings of hopelessness or pessimism; feelings of guilt, worthlessness, or helplessness; inability to concentrate, make decisions, or remember details; recurring thoughts of death or suicide, wishing to die or attempting suicide; and aches and pains, constipation, or other physical ailments that cannot be explained.

Side Effects

More common side effects may include abnormal ejaculation; abnormal vision; accidental injury; anxiety; anorexia; belching; blood in the urine; blurred vision; bronchitis; constipation; contraction of the chewing muscles; difficulty breathing; dizziness; dry mouth; ear pain; emotional swings; headache; impaired urination; impotence; inability to swallow or difficulty in swallowing; inflammation of the vagina; insomnia; lack or loss of strength; malaise; migraine; nausea; neck pain; nervousness; painful or difficult urination; prolonged drowsiness; skin discoloration; sweating; swelling of the extremities due to fluid retention; tremor; vertigo; vomiting; and weight gain.

Less common side effects may include abnormal amount of uric acid in the blood; abnormal decrease of white blood cells; abnormal protrusion of eyeball; abnormal speech; abnormal tension of arteries or muscles; absence of menstruation; allergic reaction; anemia; apathy; arthritis; asthma; attempted suicide; black stool; bladder pain; bleeding from the uterus; bone pain; bone spurs; breast pain; brittle nails; bursitis; cataract; chest congestion; chest pain; cold feet and/or hands; conjunctivitis; cornea injury; cyst; defective muscular coordination; diabetes mellitus; disease of the lymph nodes; disease of the nerves; disorder of the sense of smell; double vision; dry eyes; dry skin; enlarged abdomen; enlarged uterine fibroids; euphoria; excess of lymph cells; excessive amount of fat in the blood; excessive menstrual bleeding; excessive secretion and discharge of urine; excessive urination during the night; extreme potassium depletion; eye pain; facial swelling; generalized swelling due to fluid retention; hair loss; hallucinations; hangover effect; head tilting to one side; hemorrhoids; hernia; herpes simplex; high blood sugar; high cholesterol; hostility; hyperventilation; incoordination; increased muscular movement and physical activity; increased sensitivity to sensory stimuli; increased sex drive; increased thirst; infection of the skin or mucous membranes; inflamed prostate; inflammation of a tendon sheath, the bladder, colon, esophagus, gums, middle ear, mouth, skin, stomach and intestinal tract, or tongue; intentional injury; joint disorder; kidney pain; kidney stones; laryngitis; loss of taste; low blood pressure; low blood sugar; mouth ulceration; muscle spasm or twitching; muscular weakness and abnormal fatigue; neck rigidity; nosebleed; overdose; paranoia; pelvic pain; pneumonia; protein in the urine; psychosis; psychotic depression; pus in the urine; rash; rectal bleeding; reduced tension of arteries; sensation of numbness or tingling around the mouth; sensitivity to light; severe pain along the course of a nerve; shingles; sleep disturbance; spasm of the larynx; stomach ulcer; stupor; sugar in the urine; swelling of the tongue; temporary loss of consciousness; unusual intolerance of light; urinary incontinence; urinary urgency; vaginal bleeding; vaginal infection; visual-field defect; voice alteration; and white or yellow mucous discharge from the cervical canal or vagina.

Rare side effects may include abnormal contraction of the pupils; abnormal sensitivity to sound; abnormally colored vision; alcohol abuse; alcohol intolerance; appendicitis; bad breath; bleeding of the gums; body odor; boils; breast engorgement; breast enlargement; carcinoma; collapsed lung; complete or partial loss of muscle movement; constant and involuntary movement of the eyeballs; coughing up blood; deafness; decreased amount of protein in the blood;

decreased concentration of sodium in the blood; decreased motor reaction to stimulus; decreased pupil reflex; deficiency of oxygen; deficiency of pigmentation of the skin; deficient amount of menstrual flow; delusions; eczema; enlarged thyroid; excessive amount of potassium in the blood; excessive growth of hair; extreme slowness of movement; gallstones; glaucoma; gout; hair discoloration; hepatitis; hyperthyroidism; hypothyroidism; impairment of the ability to communicate through speech, writing, or signs; inability to sit still; increased reflexes, salivation, or sputum; infection of the mouth; inflammation of a nerve, the cornea, edges of the eyelids, gallbladder, lip, rectum and anus, the tissue that covers the white of the eye; intestinal blockage; irregular heartbeat; lactation; loss of consciousness; low blood sugar; menopause; miscarriage; osteoporosis; peptic ulcer; prolonged erection; prolonged muscle contractions; psoriasis; pustular rash; skin atrophy; slow heartbeat; soft stools; stroke; swelling of the optic nerve; temporary cessation of breathing during sleep; tongue discoloration; ulcer; ulcer of the esophagus; uterine spasm; varicose veins; vomiting of blood; withdrawal syndrome; and yellowing of the skin and whites of the eyes.

If you experience any of these side effects or reactions, notify your doctor as soon as possible.

Important Precautions

Serious, sometimes fatal, reactions have resulted from taking venlafaxine with another type of antidepressant called a monoamine oxidase inhibitor (MAOI), and when venlafaxine therapy is discontinued and MAOI therapy is started. Never take venlafaxine with one of these drugs or within two weeks of ending treatment with one of these drugs. In addition, allow at least seven days between stopping venlafaxine and starting an MAOI.

Do not take venlafaxine if you have ever had an allergic reaction or hypersensitivity to it or a similar drug.

Use this medication with caution if you have a history of kidney or liver disease, mania, seizures, or anorexia.

Venlafaxine has been associated with a sustained rise in blood pressure. For this reason, it is important to have your blood pressure monitored regularly throughout treatment with the drug.

This medication may also make you feel dizzy and drowsy. Do not drive, operate machinery, or participate in any high-risk activities until you know exactly how the drug affects you.

If you develop a skin rash, hives, or a related allergic reaction while taking venlafaxine, inform your doctor immediately.

Food and Drug Interactions

If venlafaxine is taken with certain other drugs, the effects of either drug could be increased, decreased, or changed. Before beginning treatment with venlafaxine, tell your doctor if you are taking any other prescription or over-the-counter medications.

Venlafaxine should not be combined with MAOIs. It is also important to check with your doctor before combining venlafaxine with cimetidine (Tagamet) and drugs that act on the central nervous system.

Do not drink alcohol while taking venlafaxine.

Recommended Dosage

Usual dosage for adults: The usual starting dose is 75 mg a day taken with food in two or three divided doses. This amount may be increased by 75 mg increments to a maximum of 225 mg a day for moderately depressed individuals. The severely depressed may require 350 or 375 mg a day.

The safety and effectiveness of venlafaxine use in children under the age of eighteen has not been established.

Overdosage

Symptoms of a venlafaxine overdose may include convulsions, prolonged drowsiness, and slightly increased heart rate. If you experience any of these symptoms, go to the nearest hospital emergency room immediately.

Pregnancy and Lactation

The safety of venlafaxine use during pregnancy has not been established. As a result, it should only be taken during pregnancy if the potential benefits clearly outweigh any potential risks to the fetus. If you are pregnant or plan to become pregnant, notify your doctor immediately.

Venlafaxine may pass into breast milk and may be harmful to a nursing infant. If the medication is essential to your health, your doctor may advise you not to breast-feed while you are taking it.

Zolpidem

Brand Name

Ambien

General Information

Zolpidem is a sleeping pill prescribed for the short-term treatment of insomnia. It is a member of a new class of drugs called imidazopyridines, which work by facilitating the action of the neurotransmitter GABA (gamma-aminobutyric acid). This leads to sedation, sleep, and relaxation of the large skeletal muscles.

Insomnia may involve difficulty falling asleep, waking up frequently during the night, or waking up early and not being able to get back to sleep.

Side Effects

More common side effects may include abdominal pain; abnormal dreaming; abnormal vision; amnesia; confusion; daytime drowsiness; defective muscular coordination; depression; diarrhea; dizziness; double vision; drugged feeling; dry mouth; euphoria; fatigue; headache; insomnia; lethargy; light-headedness; nausea; painful digestion; tenderness or pain in the muscles; upper respiratory infection; vertigo; and vomiting.

Less common side effects may include agitation; allergy; altered taste; anorexia; anxiety; arthritis; back pain; bronchitis; cerebrovascular disorder; chest pain; constipation; coughing; decrease in blood pressure upon standing; decreased cognition; difficult and defective speech; difficulty breathing; difficulty concentrating; dulled sensitivity to touch; emotional swings; excessive gas; eye irritation; falling; fever; flulike symptoms; hallucinations; hiccups; high blood pressure; high blood sugar; inability to swallow or difficulty in swallowing; increased sweating; infection; inflammation of the bladder, pharynx, sinuses, stomach and intestinal tract, vagina; joint pain; lack or loss of strength; malaise; menstrual disorder; migraine; nervousness; paleness; palpitation; rapid heartbeat; rash; rhinitis; ringing in the ears; sensation of numbness or tingling; severe itching; sleep disorder; stupor; swelling due to fluid retention; tooth disorder; trauma; tremor; urinary incontinence; and urinary tract infection.

Rare side effects may include abnormal decrease of white blood cells; abnormal liver function; abnormal secretion and discharge of tears; abnormal thinking; abscesses; acne; acute kidney failure; aggravated allergies; aggravated hypertension; aggression; altered salivation; anaphylactic shock (a life-threatening allergic reaction typically affecting the cardiovascular system, respiratory tract, gastrointestinal tract, and skin); anemia; belching; boils; breast pain; breast tumor or growth; bronchial spasm; circulatory failure; decreased sex drive; delusions; dementia; disease of the lymph nodes; disease of the nerves; eye pain; facial swelling; feeling of unreality; feeling strange; fluid in the lungs; flushing; frequent urination; glaucoma; gout; heart attack; hemorrhoids; herpes simplex; high cholesterol; hot flashes; hysteria; illusion; impotence; increased appetite; increased lipids in the blood; increased tolerance for the drug; inflammation of a nerve, tendon, vein, artery; inflammation of the external auditory canal, intestines, middle ear, skin, or stomach; intestinal blockage; intoxicated feeling; irregular heartbeat; joint disease; laryngitis; leg cramps; low blood pressure; manic reaction; muscle spasms; muscle weakness; neurosis; nosebleed; oxygen deficiency; pain; painful or difficult urination; panic attack; partial paralysis; persistent desire to empty the bowel or bladder; personality disorder; pneumonia; rectal bleeding; rectal pain; restless legs; sciatica; sensation of sparks or flashes of light; sensitivity to light; severe pain along the course of a nerve; shingles; skin discoloration; sleepwalking; spasm of the esophagus; speech impairment; sudden chill with high temperature followed by a sense of heat and profuse perspiration; suicide attempt; temporary loss of consciousness; thirst; tooth decay; ulceration of the cornea; urinary retention; varicose veins; weight loss; and yawning.

If you experience any of these side effects or reactions, notify your doctor as soon as possible.

Important Precautions

Do not take zolpidem if you have ever had an allergic reaction or hypersensitivity to it or a similar drug.

Use this medication with caution if you are over the age of sixty-five or physically run-down, if you have kidney or liver damage, if you suffer from depression, or if you have breathing difficulties.

The dose of zolpidem that you take at night may make you drowsy and impair your coordination the next day. Do not drive, operate machinery, or participate in any high-risk activities until you know exactly how the drug affects you.

Zolpidem is potentially addictive even when used for a relatively short time. Consequently, you may experience withdrawal symptoms when you stop taking it. Typical withdrawal symptoms include mild, temporary insomnia or irritability. Sometimes, however, more serious withdrawal symptoms such as abdominal and muscle cramps, convulsions, sweating, tremors, and vomiting occur. To help prevent withdrawal symptoms, do not abruptly discontinue zolpidem. Instead, follow your doctor's schedule for a gradual tapering of the dosage.

Food and Drug Interactions

If zolpidem is taken with certain other drugs, the effects of either drug could be increased, decreased, or changed. Before beginning treatment with zolpidem, tell your doctor if you are taking any other prescription or over-the-counter medications.

Do not drink alcohol while taking zolpidem. This combination could result in dangerously slowed breathing or coma.

For the same reason, it is important to avoid combining zolpidem with any other medications that might slow the functioning of the central nervous system, including anticonvulsants, antihistamines, antipsychotics, barbiturates, monoamine oxidase inhibitors, narcotics, or sedatives.

Recommended Dosage

Usual dosage for adults: 10 mg at bedtime.
Usual dosage for elderly or debilitated individuals: 5 mg at bedtime.

The safety and effectiveness of zolpidem use in children under the age of eighteen has not been established.

Overdosage

Symptoms of a zolpidem overdose may include coma, depressed breathing, and drowsiness. If you experience any of these symptoms, go to the nearest hospital emergency room immediately.

Pregnancy and Lactation

Zolpidem should only be taken during pregnancy if the potential benefits clearly outweigh any potential risks to the fetus. If you are pregnant or plan to become pregnant, notify your doctor immediately.

The drug passes into breast milk and may be harmful to a nursing infant. As a result, it should not be taken while breast-feeding.

Index

(See inside back cover for a cross-referenced list
of drugs by generic name)

Index

Index

Index

Index

About the Authors

Lewis A. Opler, M.D., Ph.D. is Clinical Professor of Psychiatry at Columbia University College of Physicians and Surgeons, Special Adjunct Research Professor in the Department of Psychology at Long Island University, and Medical Director of the New York City Region of the New York State Office of Mental Health.

After receiving his B.A. from Harvard University in 1969 (graduating magna cum laude in Biochemical Sciences), Dr. Opler received his Ph.D. in 1975 (in Pharmacology) and his M.D. in 1976 at the Albert Einstein College of Medicine (AECOM). Dr. Opler subsequently completed his residency in psychiatry in 1979, also at AECOM.

A significant contributor in the areas of psychopharmacology and of phenomenology, and an advocate for the rights of the severely and persistently mentally ill, Dr. Opler has been an Honorary Member of the Alliance for the Mentally Ill of New York State since 1991.

Dr. Opler was named one of the The Best Doctors in New York in *New York Magazine* in both 1991 and 1996.

Carol Bialkowski is a New Jersey–based writer who specializes in health-related topics. Her work has appeared in more than a dozen national magazines, including *American Baby, First for Women, Healthy Kids, Weight Watchers, Woman's Day, Working Mother,* and *Working Woman.* She holds a bachelor of arts degree in communication from Seton Hall University and is a member of the American Society of Journalists and Authors.

THE PDR
POCKET GUIDE
TO PRESCRIPTION DRUGS

*Based on Physicians' Desk Reference®,
the Nation's Leading Professional Drug Handbook*

♦ Complete, Unabridged and Up-to-Date
Drug Listings from *The PDR Family Guide to
Prescription Drugs*®

♦ Quick, Easy Alphabetical Reference by
Familiar Brand Names—with Convenient
Generic Cross-Reference

♦ Plus: 32 Pages of Color Photographs of the
Most Common Drugs

NOW AVAILABLE FROM POCKET BOOKS